# Psycho-Spiritual Healing

*And Other Techniques for Dysfunctions Created by Who We Are and How We Incarnate*

By

Guy Steven Needler

2nd-2022



Library of Congress Cataloging-in-Publication Data

Guy Steven Needler – 1961-

*Psycho-Spiritual Healing* by Guy Steven Needler

*Psycho-Spiritual Healing* describes the various healing modalities used in treating, physical, energetic and psycho-spiritual issues.

1. Spiritual 2. Healing 3. Energies 4. Modalities
I. Guy Steven Needler, 1961 II. Metaphysical III. Healing IV. Title

Library of Congress Catalog Card Number: 2020950639
ISBN: 9781940265933

Cover Art and Layout: Victoria Cooper Art
Book set in: Times New Roman and Schnebel Sans Pro Comp.
Book Design: Summer Garr
Published by:

OZARK MOUNTAIN PUBLISHING

PO Box 754, Huntsville, AR 72740
800-935-0045 or 479-738-2348; fax 479-738-2448
WWW.OZARKMT.COM

Printed in the United States of Americ

# Table of Contents

**Illustrations by Nina Špolar "nini"**

# Books by Guy Needler

The History of God
Published by: Ozark Mountain Publishing

Beyond the Source, Book One
Published by: Ozark mountain Publishing

Beyond the Source, Book Two
Published by: Ozark Mountain Publishing

Avoiding Karma
Published by: Ozark Mountain Publishing

The Origin Speaks
Published by: Ozark Mountain Publishing

The Anne Dialogues
Published by: Ozark Mountain Publishing

The Curators
Published by: Ozark Mountain Publishing

OZARK
MOUNTAIN
PUBLISHING

For more information about any of the above titles, soon to be released titles, or other items in our catalog, write, phone or visit our website:
Ozark Mountain Publishing, Inc.
PO Box 754, Huntsville, AR 72740
479-738-2348/800-935-0045
www.ozarkmt.com

# Foreword

This book, at first glance, would appear to be a departure from my usual subject matter. However, when one considers that everything I have written to date was initiated by me enrolling in a healing workshop in 2001 presented by Helen Stott, a direct student of Barbara Brennan, previously a NASA scientist, who used channeling to establish more information about the patient the healer was working on, you should be able to see the link. The origin of the energy and vibrational healing is therefore based upon the teachings of Barbara Brennan, which were subsequently taught to me over four years by Helen. This is my heritage and lineage.

My reentry into the multiverse was initially supported by me opening a small healing practice in a holistic venue close to my home in 2005. This floundered at best and then failed, resulting in me focusing upon the information I gained through channeling rather than the healing itself, which disappeared into the background. Later, when The History of God was written in 2010, I created a website to support its Internet visibility and felt drawn to offer channeling-based readings and of course the energy and vibrational healing I was taught by Helen via the same website. One by one, I started to receive requests for both readings and healings from people all over the world, all possible by the use of Skype, QQ, WhatsApp, and WeChat. Together with channeling more books and creating the Traversing the Frequencies workshops, the rest is history, so to speak.

Although I initially worked within the framework of those techniques I studied, I found that I was accessing other techniques or modalities that were new and not currently available, creating new modalities of healing and adding them to my repertoire. My communications with The Source were allowing me to create both new and bespoke healing modalities required for all or one patient only. Additionally, my late wife, Anne, has helped me at times as well, making important suggestions about healing requirements and possibilities.

As I worked on a plethora of different patients (from literally all over the world), I noticed that some of the bespoke modalities could also be generalized allowing many others to benefit from me working on the illness of one. I also noticed that much of what we bring into this incarnation, including our method of incarnation, affects us energetically creating physical dysfunction through psycho-spiritual programming.

Having perfected these techniques and using them with, in some cases, miraculous success, I felt a very strong need to share this work, via a book, with the wider spiritual public. I do have to say though that this book is not supposed to detract one from attending a fully certified healing workshop or school, but is designed to show some level of detail and act as a trigger for those who want to be a healer, to see what the art of the possible is, and to seek proper tuition. Please note that some people are not meant to be healed, that their illness is part of their incarnate experience, or their way out of this incarnation. It is part of the role of the healer to recognize this, providing assistance and not a cure, not engaging the ego or the determined healer thinking, "YOU WILL BE HEALED—SO HELP ME GOD!"

I strongly advocate that the budding healer goes through an essential program of psycho-analytical work to assist in cleaning and clearing the psyche and distancing one from one's ego while undergoing training. This will help to ensure that one's "stuff" is not passed on to the patient and the patient's "stuff" is not received by the healer. I will be recommending some authors and books to use to get you started. Healing can be deeply searching from the psychological perspective and is not for the fainthearted.

I said that I would give some level of detail to the

modalities I will be describing, and in most instances it will be very detailed and may look like it is instructional. However, when you go to a healer, check to see where they gained their qualifications, that they received instruction from a recognized course and have not just gained academic knowledge from a book.

In your reading of this book, I am illustrating to you what I do, and how I do it, not teaching you per se. I am simply opening you up to your healing potential and some of the things that can be done.

I have noted over the years that healing and my healing modalities are sometimes aligned to each other in a genre of healing, and sometimes they are not but are more standalone. As a result, this book will be presented in five main genres. The healing modalities I use fall into:

1. Energy and Vibrational Healing, including work on the chakras and entity removal
2. Removing Links—links with other incarnates, non-karmic and karmic, plus individual karma and past life trauma
3. Client-Based or Bespoke Healing—mixtures of different healing modalities together
4. Psycho-Spiritual Reprogramming, removal of deep-rooted thoughts, behaviors, and actions
5. How We Incarnate and How It Affects Us Psychologically: Psychosis

The details behind these major genres will be presented as chapters within them.

Additionally, I would like to make a comment on the way I address the patient/client and the healer. There are times when I address the healer as "the healer" and others where I address the healer as "you." The use of "you" can also be used to reference "himself/herself." Similarly, there are times when I address the client or patient as the "patient" or "client" and others when I use "they." This is designed to give "you" the reader a focus on the fact that you may, or may not be, a healer per se, but are simply interested in this particular aspect of the greater reality. Also note that "they" can also be used to reference "he/she."

Please note that the illustrations are conceptual and may change with the psycho-spiritual and intuitive visualization capability (experiential vocabulary) of the healer.

Guy Steven Needler
June 2018

# General Notes Prior to Performing a Healing

In general, a form should be employed indicating the process of the healing and expected physical sensations together with permission or authority for the healer to perform the healing in the form of a signature from the client before starting the healing. Similar concurrence can be gained by the use of a tick box on the healer's website if payment via the website is made or concurrence by use of the payment system provided a note of acceptance is located in an obvious position close to the payment system on the website itself.

The healer should first employ the use of a good-quality therapy couch. It should be placed in a room dedicated to the healer's therapy and positioned so that there is plenty of room to move around the couch with a chair with castor wheels if necessary. I prefer to heal sitting down; it is a comfortable position to be in and if the healer is comfortable then the client will have a comfortable energetic experience.

Any energies from previous clients can be cleared from the room by smudging the air by burning incense.

# Preliminary Consultation / Normal Consultation

Before starting any healing modality and indeed during the first meeting between the healer and the patient, it is advisable to perform a short fifteen- to twenty-minute consultation. Subsequent consultations may be shorter. The first consultation may require what is normally a one-hour appointment to be one hour fifteen minutes to allow an appropriate length of time for the healing process. Please be advised that any notes that are taken are classified as private/confidential and should therefore be stored in an appropriate and safe area.

During the consultation the healer should ask a number of questions of the patient to help him/her ascertain the modality/ies of healing necessary and more importantly the origin of the issue/s that caused the physical manifestations or psycho-spiritual issues that are required to be healed. These questions can be illustrated by the following subjects:

- Feelings
- Emotions
- Past memories (not experiences)
- Frustrations
- Physical pain and its location
- Psychological issues such as anxiety, depression, etc.
- Fears

- Interaction with others
- Likes and dislikes
- Food eaten
- Accidents
- Recent experiences
- Past experiences (not memories)
- Links with family, friends, and work colleagues

Through asking questions based upon these subjects, the healer, in using his/her intuition, can create a picture of where the underlying issues were manifest and what modality or combination of modalities should be employed to effect a healing.

Once you have established the modality/ies of healing to be employed, the healer should gain authority from the patient to move into their energies, which should include the advice that you may place your hands on the areas of chelation within this authority. You are now ready to perform a healing. Please note that it may be appropriate to cover the patient's body with a warm blanket to help them stay warm.

Once I have established, through a combination of analysis and intuition, what type/s or modalities of healings are required to be performed on the client, I advise them what I am going to do and explain why I am going to do it.

# Energy and Vibrational Healing: Natural Healing Using Nature's Basic Principles

## What Is Energy and Vibrational Healing?

Energy and vibrational healing is a gentle noninvasive therapy and covers a plethora of minor modalities such as Reiki, Brennan Healing Science, and other hands-on healing techniques, including those that are unregulated. It does not cover the usage of an intermediate focus of the energies channeled by the healer such as the use of pendulums, stones, crystals, acupuncture, acupressure, candles, or other physical interfaces. It heals the physical manifestation of dis-ease, which results from imbalances in the human energy field and the energetic templates that allow the manifestation of the gross physical aspect of the human body we incarnate into. In most cases these imbalances are created by misperceptions of events encountered during our early years of life that are reflected on the body's energy system. These ultimately create physical dis-ease and dysfunction. However, they can be caused by other things such as how we incarnate, what we bring into this incarnation from a previous incarnation, and how addicted we are to the low frequency thoughts, behaviors, and actions associated with incarnating into a low frequency environment. This is called karma and will be dealt with in its own chapter.

Because I mentioned physical interfaces above, I feel a need to explain a few things about them. A physical interface is a method used to provide the healer, or indeed a channeler, with a focus, or even confidence that they can do that which they want to do while using the physical interface of choice or that is aligned to the modality of healing they are specialized in.

So, those that use them subconsciously feel that they can only effect a healing when they use them. Indeed, the use of such physical interfaces is limited to the energies they are associated with and so limits the ability of the healer to provide a holistic healing service. This is not to say that those who specialize in healing modalities that require a physical interface are poor practitioners, it is just that they are specialized in a certain healing modality, one that requires the use of the focus of the physical interface they are trained in or drawn to use. They are not holistic and generally cannot heal issues that fall outside the capabilities of their specialism. If they do manage to heal an issue outside of the capabilities of their specialism, it is because they are subconsciously using another modality which may be being channeled through them at the behest of the collaboration between the Guide and Helpers of the client and the healer.

Energy and vibrational healing usually requires light placement of the practitioner's hands over different areas of the client's body; it is not a physical interface but a way of affecting a direct method of channeling energy from the healer to the client. Note, however, that the energy is not actually from the healer but is channeled through the healer from the free energies that pervade The Source Entity, our creator. The hands can be placed a few centimeters above the client if desired. It is normally carried out with the client lying on a therapy table, in order to promote good relaxation but can be and is also performed at a distance (distance or absence healing) with the same level of success. A session may leave the client feeling in a rather different state than usual, so that it is best not to move or animate the body quickly or drive immediately after a healing.

## What Are the Healing Techniques Used?

There are a number of healing techniques that can be employed during the healing process and some of these are mentioned below:

- Chelation (basic energy balancing)
- Chakra reconstruction
- Organ reconstruction
- Psychic surgery
- Auric-level reconstruction
- Astral entity removal
- Astral mucus clearing
- Virus clearing
- Spine cleansing
- Brain balancing
- Hara Line healing
- Foreign object removal

Other healing modalities that I use that are not mentioned above will be noted in their own chapters because I feel they are not specifically related to the genre of energy and vibrational healing.

## Chelation (basic energy balancing)

Chelation is the most basic of healing techniques and also the most benign. It is simple and easy to perform and requires little if no actual complicated interaction with the client by the healer.

Chelation is a healing technique where the healer places the hands over specific areas of the gross physical body allowing the divine energies of The Source to be channeled through the healer without intervention.

There are sixteen points of contact/no contact that are used to channel healing energies during the chelation-based healing. They are:

1. The left ankle
2. The right ankle
3. The left knee
4. The right knee
5. The left hip
6. The right hip
7. The front aspect of the sacral chakra
8. The front aspect of the solar chakra
9. The front apsect of the heart chakra
10. The left shoulder
11. The right shoulder
12. The front aspect of the throat chakra
13. The rear aspect of the throat chakra
14. The left-hand temple area of the head
15. The right-hand temple area of the head
16. The crown chakra

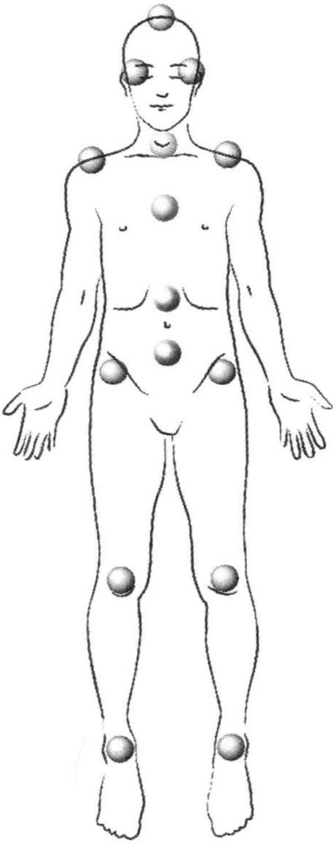

Note that I only specified the front aspects of the sacral, solar, and heart chakras. (See the next chapter on chakra regeneration for the locations of the chakras.) This is because the horizontal chakras have psycho-spiritual functions are well. The front chakra is our intention and the rear chakra is our action so whatever we do or request of the front chakras the rear chakras receive or do automatically. However, some healers performing chelation do place the hands over both the front and rear aspects of the sacral, solar, and heart chakras during chelation. Also note that the spiritual or third eye chakras are not used. I will explain the process of performing a chelation in full now.

## How to Perform a Chelation

Chelation is performed by the use of placing the hand, palm opened, on the area of the position of the chelation. The palm of the hand is the position of a minor chakra.

The length of time spent in one position within the chelation-based healing is a function of the healer's intuition, but I have found that it is usual to stay for between two to three minutes in each position. Using the chelation points previously stated, I usually place the palms of my hands in the following combinations of positions:

Note that the position of the healer in relation to the patient is a function of personal choice and comfort.

1. The left and right ankles
2. The left ankle and left knee
3. The left knee and left hip
4. The right ankle and right knee
5. The right knee and right hip
6. The right and left hips
7. The left hip and front aspect of the sacral chakra (can be just front and rear aspects of the chakra)
8. The front aspect of the sacral chakra and the front aspect of the solar chakra (can be just the front and rear aspects of the chakra)
9. The front aspect of the solar chakra and the front aspect of the heart chakra (can be just the front and rear aspects of the chakra)
10. The front aspect of the heart chakra and the left shoulder
11. The left and right shoulders

12. The right shoulder and the front aspect of the throat chakra
13. The front and rear aspects of the throat chakra
14. The left- and the right- hand temples are of the head. The hands should be placed just above the ears with the third and fourth fingers either side of the ears.
15. The crown chakra; the right hand should be over the crown chakra with the left hand on top of the right hand.
16. When you feel that the healing is completed, move out of the energy field of your client and visualize resealing it. This recreates the integrity of the seven layers of the human energy field and reestablishes its normal protective properties.

Example of the Chelation Points and Position of the Healer

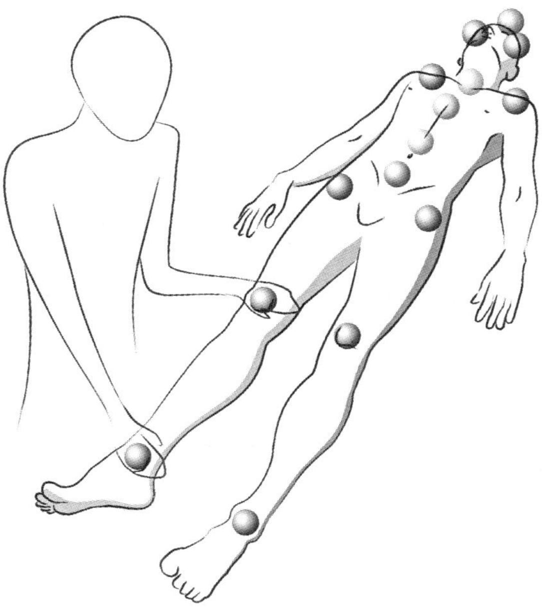

## Explanation of Performing Distance Chelation

As I stated in the foreword, a lot of the healing work I perform is "distance-based." This means I am in communication with the client via some form of video telephony such as Skype, WhatsApp, QQ, or We Chat or simply an audio telephone (landline or mobile/cell phone).

When I perform these distance-based healings, I use the exact same process that I would use when performing a "physical" presence-based healing. However, for the client, this is not what I would call value for money as they would be either sitting or lying down on a bed or couch in their home or other quiet and private location and not be experiencing anything else from a physical perspective.

Remember we are incarnate into a physical vehicle and therefore desire physical feedback of some sort most of the time. This is true no matter how spiritually aligned we are.

In order to address this problem, I do three things.

1. I advise the clients that they may experience certain physical sensation-based phenomena and that they should look out for such reactions within themselves during the healing process. I don't advise them what they would be because this would create expectation and distract them from the potential to experience the plethora of sensations that they may experience through focusing on the one that they would "like" or "prefer" to experience. Suffice to say these sensations can be experienced as heat, tingling, pressure around the area of the third eye, the crown of the head, or the periphery of the skull, tinnitus, visualizations in the closed-eye vision, and energy movements within the body or emotional content.

2. I explain what I am doing as I do it. I feel that in distance-based healing this is important as it involves the client's own visualization process of the healing as it is being performed creating a synergetic effect that augments the effectivity of the healing being administered.

3. I make an audio recording of the healing and send it to the clients. Giving the clients an audio recording of the healing is important because they can review, in the privacy of their own home, what they have received from a healing perspective. Additionally, placing themselves in a comfortable position while listening to the recording of their healing places them in the same "Event Space" as that experienced when receiving the "real-time" healing. This is of significant benefit to the clients from both a healing and a financial perspective. Indeed, I have had many clients advise me that they received all of the same sensations experienced when in the real-time healing. I do not believe that these are just psychosomatic or placebo-based responses but are very real and very beneficial.

4. Note that I do not retain copies of the recordings of my clients' healings. I see the recordings as the sole property of the clients and this practice helps to maintain their privacy. I also do not condone the audio of the healing being uploaded onto social media by clients. I have the same policy for audio recordings of readings.

# Chakra Reconstruction

## What Are the Chakras?

The chakras can basically be described as energy junctures. They are distributed around the human body at various points where the energy distribution lines meet or are joined together. They come in three main sizes, major, minor, and mini. The major and minor chakras are the most important from a healing perspective with the major chakras usually needing to be healed in some way and the minor chakras in the palms of the hands being used for healing during chelation.

The flow of energy in the minor chakras of the hands is usually pushed out from the palms to the point or area required to be healed. The flow should be natural and not "pushed" as pushing the energies into a patient can be detrimental to the healing process and uses the ego of the healer to heal in a certain and successful way rather than the patient's desire to be healed, the healer being a simple interface with the healing energy of The Source and The Source itself.

The minor chakras can also be used in psychometry. Psychometry is the sensing of an object's use or history by linking into its natural energies by the use of the chakras in the hands.

When I talk about chakra reconstruction, therefore, I talk about the healing of the front and rear aspects of the major chakras only. First, though, I will discuss the construction of the major chakras.

## Anatomy of a Chakra

The major chakras are described and illustrated in many and varying ways in numerous spiritual texts and artwork. They range from the factual to the wholly inaccurate in both their description and illustration. I have therefore come to recognize that the level of description and illustration is a function of the level of education of the writer, healer, or illustrator. I also note a secondary function of when the text/illustration was written/drawn, the era the work was done in, and the world spatial location.

Without a doubt in my mind, the descriptions of both Hindu texts and the observational illustrations of Barbara Brennan provide the most accurate information on the size, shape, and functionality of the chakras to date.

The best way to understand what a chakra is then is to study the Hindu texts and the works of Barbara Brennan (see ***Hands of Light*** and ***Light Emerging***). Having pointed out the locations for you to find the best information, it would be remiss of me to not summarize this information for you.

The major chakras are energy receptors that work on the first seven frequency levels associated with the physical universe. The human body uses the energies of the first ten frequency levels of the physical universe to create and maintain/sustain it. Levels 1–7 support the integration of the sentient energy of the Aspect or Soul with the human body and levels 8–10 provide the energetic "step-down" function that allows the compression of the communicative bandwidth and allows the Aspect or Soul itself to enter into levels 1–7, which are necessary for incarnation in the gross physical.

The chakras "pull" energy "in" to assist in the incarnate Aspect or Soul's maintenance and animation of the gross physical (frequency levels 1–3) and spirituo-physical aspects of the human body (frequency levels 4–7). They are cone-shaped, vortex-based receptors that have a number of minor vortex-based receptors within them. They are like vortices within the overall form of the vortex of the chakra. Each of the chakras is frequentially associated with the energy template that creates the human body of the same frequency, 1–7. The use of these energies by the chakras creates a form of radiation associated with the first seven frequency levels. This is called the human aura or human energy field.

All of the major chakras are joined together via a main energy conduit, which is ultimately co-joined to the Hara Line. The Hara Line is that tube of energy that protects the sentient energy of the Aspect or Soul allowing it to enter into the construct of the human body and maintain some form of communicative capability with the True Energetic Self (TES). Although, the communicative bandwidth is drastically reduced as a function of moving down into the frequencies that necessitate incarnation to interact with a low frequency environment, some communication is still possible and the incarnate Aspect or Soul is never actually disconnected from the TES.

The number of smaller vortices within a chakra is specific to the overall number of subfrequencies within a frequency level. The lower the frequencies a chakra has to work with, the lower the number of smaller vortices that are within it. The higher the frequencies a chakra has to work with, the higher the number of smaller vortices that are within it. For example, the base or root chakra has a low number of smaller vortices within it due to the low number, fewer than ten, of subfrequencies. On the other hand, the crown chakra has a high number of smaller vortices within it due to the high number, hundreds, of subfrequencies.

The chakras therefore work on a complicated broadband spectrum of subfrequencies within the overall frequency levels that they are associated with. All of these frequencies and subfrequencies are needed to assure a complete integration of the Aspect or Soul with the human body allowing the command and control, the animation of, the human body by the sentient energy of the Aspect or Soul in a seamless way. In the correct high frequency environment, the energy of the frequencies received by the chakras is all that is necessary to sustain and perpetuate the existence of the human body as a useful vehicle for interacting with a low frequency environment of a level that is higher than that experienced by us all now. However, due to the preceding and current frequency levels being very low at best, it is necessary to consume the energy associated with vegetables, fruits, berries, nuts, pulses, and fungi. Hence our need and desire to eat and drink. Although certain blood groups are predisposed to being vegetarian (herbivore), meat-eating (carnivorous), or need both physical foods (omnivorous), with correct training a person can still sustain his or her human body by energy alone.

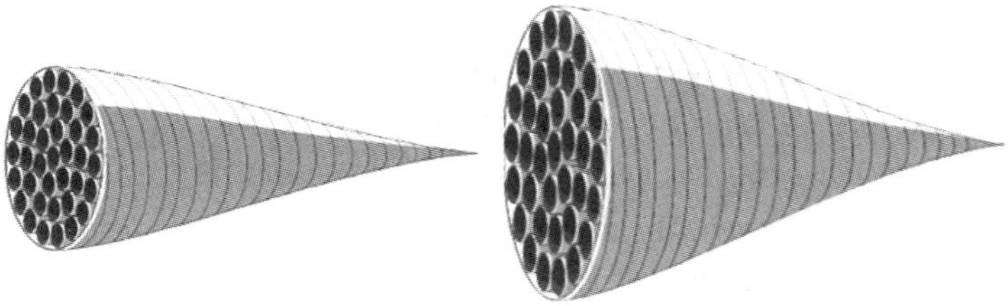

Basic illustration of a Chakra (one more open [larger] than the other)
Here the internal vortices can be seen.

## Why the Chakras Need Repair or Reconstruction

As well as being used for energy reception to maintain the incarnate human body, the chakras are also used in the many ways we have of communicating energetically. As a result of being used for other purposes the chakras are exposed to being damaged or abused. Damage and abuse can result in the failure or reduced function or efficiency of a chakra, which ultimately creates physical dysfunction and illness. These can be described in the categories below:

**Psychological and emotional issues within the self** are created by how we are programmed by our parents, teachers, peers, environment, and overall incarnate experience.

Psychological and emotional issues create a condition where the balanced use of a chakra is disturbed to the point where certain frequencies are ignored, not desired, overdesired, or rejected. The effect on the operational functions of the chakras in this way further supports the psychological or emotional issues that are being experienced, creating a downward spiral in both the chakras and the individual. The visual appearance of the chakra / chakras concerned varies but in general it can be seen that certain vortices within the chakra are either inflamed, atrophied, nonfunctional, oversized, or abnormal in shape. In each case described, an internal chakra vortex that displays one of these visual attributes will need to be replaced by the healer. See the table below this text for the psychological functions of the chakras.

**Psychological and emotional issues between people** are created by how we interact on a one-to-one basis with certain individuals rather than being general programming issues.

Psychological and emotional issues between people also create a condition where the balanced use of a chakra is disturbed to the point where certain frequencies are ignored, not desired, overdesired, or rejected, creating similar or the same visual appearances as those described above. The interesting point to note here is that the chakras may recover when the issues between the people concerned are either resolved or removed through lack of association or the removal of a link or karmic link. It is also possible that the chakras may change to the dysfunctional state only when interacting with the individual/s of concern so the healer may need to refer to a psycho-spiritual or link removal approach rather than healing the chakras per se. However, if the dysfunctional state is maintained outside of the interaction with the individual/s concerned then the vortices will need to be replaced together with psycho-spiritual reprogramming (see the chapter on psycho-spiritual reprogramming later in this book).

**Psychological Function of Chakras and Name, Appearance, and Function of the Auric Layers / Energy Levels**

| | Chakra | Chakra | |
|---|---|---|---|
| | | "Front" Action | "Rear" Action |
| ☀ | Root | Quantity of physical energy, will to live | |
| ☀ | Sacral | Quality of love for the opposite sex, giving and receiving mental and spiritual pleasure. | Quality of sexual energy. |
| ☀ | Solar | Pleasure and expansiveness, spiritual wisdom, consciousness of the universality of life and who you are in the universe. | Healing and intentionality toward your health |
| ☀ | Heart | Heart feelings of love toward other human beings, openness to life | Ego, will, or will toward the outer world. |
| ☀ | Throat | Taking in and assimilating knowledge | Sense of self within society and one's profession |
| ☀ | Spiritual Eye | Copacity to visualize and understand mental concepts | Ability to acheive ideas in a practical way |
| ☀ | Crown | Integration of personality with life and spiritual aspects of mankind | |

Adapted from Barbara Brennan, Hands of Light (Bantam Books, 1987), Fig. 9-1, p. 73.

**An energetic attack** on an individual's energy body, body, chakra, or chakras can be a conscious, unconscious, specific, general, or collective (more than one person involved) act. Depending upon the issues surrounding the desire to attack an individual, the energies and frequencies from one or more chakras can be used by the assailant to attack another. Based upon this, it can be understood that the chakras can be used to project energy as well as receive energy. (The direction of rotation creates the push or pull of energy/frequency.)

An energy attack on the chakras can damage the whole chakra, demanding major reconstruction or even replacement of one or a number of the vortices within the chakra. In any energy attack on the chakras, the resulting imagery received illustrates either disfigurement of the chakra or its vortices or outright burnout resulting in serious physical dysfunctional response or illness.

**Astral entity attachment** is more common than one would imagine. Astral entities are created in one of two major ways. First, they can be consciously or unconsciously created from energies in the fourth to seventh frequencies, but usually the fourth and fifth, by a specific individual and projected/directed toward the person that is being targeted as a function of anger or dislike by that individual. Second, they can be created as a natural function of evolution through the attraction of similar or same energies and the resulting creation of minor or rudimentary intelligence. Whereas astral entities that are created through an incarnate individual's anger are perpetuated in existence by that individual (should that conscious or unconscious desire remain), astral entities that are created through natural evolution are not capable of generating their own energy to perpetuate their existence and so can and do have a very transient period of cohesion in one particular state of rudimentary intelligence. As such, astral entities only maintain their individualized existence from a longer-term perspective through the energies of another, either their creator or a host. This survivability requirement, being recognized by the astral entity on a very basic level, usually motivates it to the point where it seeks out a suitable source of free energy, a host, and attaches/associates itself to the host. More often than not, the astral entity attaches itself to an area of the human body where it is not noticeable, but where it can create an energetic link to the unsuspecting host, or better still, create a synergetic dependency between the host and the astral entity where the host receives some form of power or coercive function over others.

Astral entities come in all shapes and sizes and therefore have varying levels of energetic demands on their host, who will generally feel tired, unless there is a synergetic exchange involved. When an astral entity attaches itself to a host via a chakra, usually a major chakra, it uses most of the energy and frequencies received by that chakra leaving a bare minimum to sustain the host, hence the feeling of being tired. The astral entity attaches itself to the chakra by digging or plugging itself into one or more of the vortices within the chakra, which damages that vortex and blocks the frequencies and energies being received by the others so that it can use them itself. In effect, it becomes part of the receptive function of the chakra while damaging that chakra. As a result, a chakra that has been used by an astral entity to sustain its continued existence usually needs major reconstruction or replacement once the astral entity has been removed.

Illustrations of Astral entities attacking a chakra. External and Internal attacks/attachments shown.

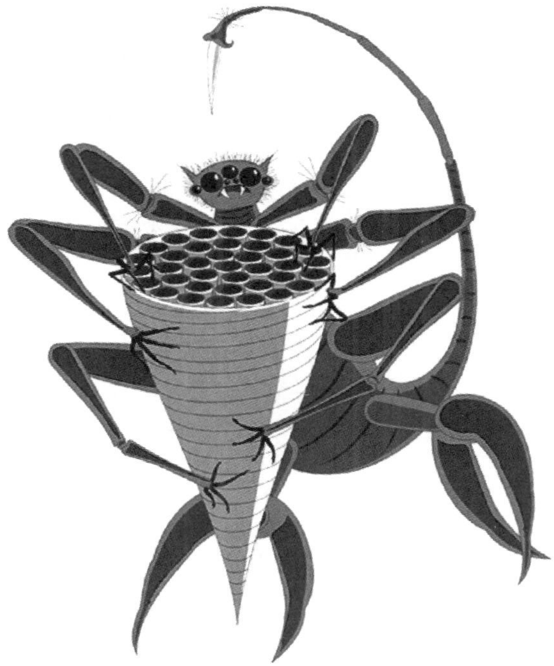

A Spider/Crab-like Entity outside the Chakra

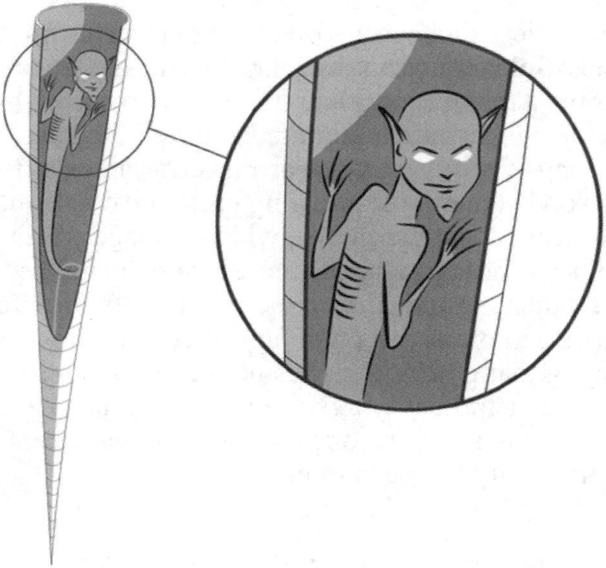

An Imp-like Entity inside a Vortex

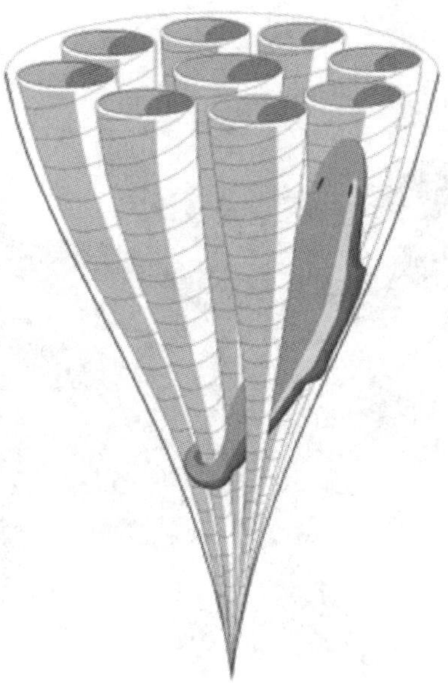

A Slug-like Entity in between the Vortices

## General Wear and Tear

One would think that energetic components of our incarnate vehicle would not be subject to general wear and tear, but they are. They are not subject to wear in normal circumstances but they are subject to wear as a result of our psycho-spiritual thought processes and actions.

Such actions are lack of proper nutrition; lack of proper exercise; dysfunctional thoughts, behaviors, and actions; poor environmental conditions; drugs and alcohol intake; overindulgence in food and exercise. There is an old saying, everything in moderation is fine but we do tend to overindulge in that which we like.

The wear-and-tear damage on the chakras associated with the gross physical is therefore created by the imbalances that were created by extreme focus on the physical, whereas wear-and-tear damage on the chakras associated with the spirituo-physical is created by the imbalances that were created by extreme focus on the metaphysical.

We need to live in balance with whom and what we are—and the fact that the incarnate vehicle is a very complex device—not just from the physical perspective but also from the energetic perspective.

Focusing on the gross physical means that we are addicted to low frequency existence while incarnate and ignore the metaphysical or spirituo-physical. Focusing on the spirituo-physical or metaphysical means that we are addicted to higher frequency existence while incarnate and ignore the gross physical.

Unbalanced incarnate existence puts a strain on those chakras that are being overused as a result of focus on one aspect of our incarnate existence and causes those chakras that are not being used to go into a state of atrophy through lack of use.

General wear and tear is an overall function of those issues that create the degradation of the efficiency of the function of the chakras over time. It ultimately results in the reconstruction or total replacement of a chakra or number of chakras to ensure the continued opportunity for incarnate existence is maintained. If reconstruction of, or replacement of, a chakra or chakras is not achieved in a timely manner then the gross physical aspect of one's incarnate vehicle will be affected detrimentally, which can and does include psychological issues.

## Low Frequency Interruption

Low frequency interruption is a condition that all chakras are exposed to, irrespective of one's ability to exist in a balanced way. Low frequency interruption is a function of existing in one's normal environment and is the result of the chakras attracting stray low frequency energy. Functioning almost like dust, this stray low frequency energy gets attracted to the chakras and the vortices within them by what can only be described as a function of the normal energy flow from the outside environment to the chakra. It is sucked into the area of the chakra by the flow of energy and covers the outside of the individual chakra vortices, the receptor area of the vortices within the chakra, and fills in the gaps in between the vortices.

With the vortices within the chakras being covered in low frequency energy, the efficiency of the chakras to pull in energy associated with that chakra is impaired resulting in a functional imbalance, which has a detrimental effect on the gross physical and spirituo-physical energetic templates that create the incarnate vehicle. This can and does result in rapid ageing of the gross physical.

## Chakra Disfigurement

Chakra disfigurement is when the normal size and shape of a chakra, its representation as a healthy chakra, is compromised as a result of any of the issues described above and below. The shape of the chakra can represent the type of stress or damage it has sustained as a result of psychic or energetic attack, skewed use, atrophy, astral entity, or foreign body attachment to the chakra. The chakra can present damaged, missing, or detached inner vortices to the healer along with abnormal external appearances. In any of these instances, the healer will need to decide whether to repair the chakra by repairing or replacing the vortices, change the outer skin (energetic shape) of the chakra as a whole, or indeed replace the whole chakra.

Descriptions on how this can be achieved are illustrated later in this chapter.

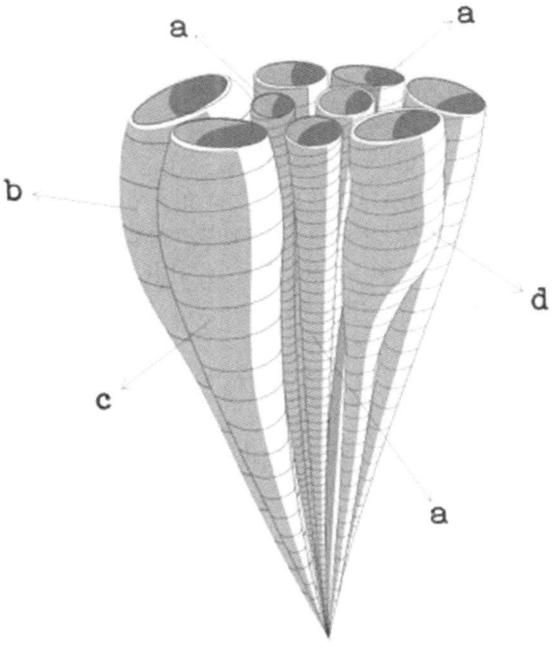


Visual Appearance of Damaged Inner Vortices That Need Repair

a) Atrophied
b) Oversized
c) Inflamed
d) Normal

## Skewed Use of a Particular Chakra or Chakra Set

Skewed use of a particular chakra or chakra set is a function of psycho-spiritual imbalance on all levels. Although over time it can be a function of general wear and tear, it can also be a function of a change in one's mental condition and can take effect on a fast or rapid basis.

There are two classifications of chakra set: the gross physical, which is associated with the base, sacral, and solar chakras, and the spirituo-physical, which is associated with the heart, throat, third eye, and crown chakras.

The skewed use of a particular chakra set is therefore attributed predominantly to being in the gross physical or in the spirituo-physical to the detriment of the other chakra set. The predominant use of one chakra set above another results in the chakra set being ignored, atrophying to the point of minor effectivity but not in total function.

Note that the functionality of the incarnate vehicle cannot be sustained if any of the chakra sets or individual chakras atrophy to the point of inaction. If they do then a terminal genetic illness is contracted and the incarnation is terminated as a result.

The skewed use of the chakra sets and individual chakras have the following physical/psycho-spiritual symptoms:

Skewed use of the **gross physical** results in the focus of the physical as the only aspect of that which one is. Physically these individuals are either lethargic or overweight or focused on physical appearance. In both cases, mental focus is on the physical such as materialism, status, and wealth, or the fact that they do not have these but others do, and bear resentment. In both conditions, the individual's incarnation is terminated early due to health issues through lack of care, poor diet, or heart attack caused by inappropriate use of body-building supplements or overexercise. Mental issues such as "poor me" syndrome may also ensue when they compare themselves to others with more material wealth.

Skewed use of the **spirituo-physical** results in the focus of the spiritual as the only aspect of that which one is. Physically these individuals are either underweight or focused on spiritual practices to the detriment of their physical body. They may even have the appearance of being "new age." They should not be confused with those who drop out of society or their responsibilities, although they can appear as such. In both cases mental focus is on the metaphysical such as being detached, superior, and feeling that they can go without physical nourishment for indefinite periods. In this condition, the individual's incarnation is terminated early again due to health issues through lack of care of the physical. Additionally, they tend to miss the point of their incarnate experience and do not fulfill their responsibilities in the gross physical environment and wonder what went wrong when their world falls apart from lack of due care and attention. The general demeanor of these people is that God (Source) will provide for them, sort out their issues, or bring them wealth, and when God doesn't—God invariably helps those who help themselves—they become distrustful and try to discredit spiritualism and spiritual people. In essence, they create the reverse of what they wanted to be.

I will make a point here of stating that focus on the spiritual, although desirable, does not relinquish one from one's everyday responsibilities or interactions associated with one's incarnation or life plan. Being spiritual means being balanced and not skewed one way or another. We are here for the purpose of accelerating our evolutionary progression through the use of being incarnate in a low frequency environment, and the wise and advanced spiritual individual knows this.

Skewed use of the **root or base chakra** results in one being highly sexually oriented. This can result in overdependence on sex and can be detrimental to one's relationship with one's partner. Promiscuity can also develop along with fetish-based sexual behavior that can be mild to extreme in activity. Sexual disease can manifest as a result in the skewed use of the root or base chakra. Physical issues associated with the spinal column and kidneys are common. Sexually transmitted diseases can also be contracted by these people. These people are generally very immersed in their incarnation.

Skewed use of the **sacral chakra** results in a want to have a family. In this instance, a high number of children within one's family, or if married more than once, "families," is indicative of a predominant use of the sacral chakra. If this want or desire is unfulfilled then issues associated with the reproductive system are likely. This can manifest in ovarian cysts, ovarian cancer, cervical cancer, and so on. These diseases may also prevail if a number of children lower than that wanted are produced. One should not confuse the effects of the skewed used of the sacral chakra with that of the base or root chakra.

Skewed use of the **solar chakra** results in a feeling that one is never full or is anxious about any issue that is felt to be out of the hands of the individual. Overdependence on the solar chakra can also create issues with the pancreas, the stomach, the circulatory functions of the liver, and the gall bladder. Issues with nervous tension can also prevail together with the associated physical responses such as uncontrollable shaking of the hands (similar to, but not the same as Parkinson's disease), or the lack of use of limbs or accelerated metabolic functions. The nervous/anxious energy generated by these people can be illustrated by them needing a lot of physical nourishment on a regular basis but never actually gaining weight.

Skewed use of the **heart chakra** psycho-spiritually results in being overly trusting from a relationship perspective and can lead to disappointments that are difficult to overcome. From the physical perspective the overall functions of the circulatory system, heart, blood, and the Vagus nerve can be overused, creating a condition where they experience age acceleration. This is specifically noted by higher than normal pulse rates and blood pressure problems. Palpitations can also be prevalent. These people usually end up with some form of heart disease or enlargement of one of the heart valves.

Skewed use of the **throat chakra** can be seen by people who are loquacious or forceful in the presentation of verbal interactions, they like to shout a lot and be heard. Physical issues with the bronchial and vocal chords, the lungs, such as with asthma, can also be observed with those who overwork this chakra. The alimentary canal may also be subject to infection. It is quite common for these people to be singers or politicians.

Skewed use of the **spiritual or third eye chakra** results in overuse of the pituitary gland and what can be described as spiritual "black out." Although the spiritual or third eye is one of the most fundamental tools one can use in spiritual functionality, overuse of the spiritual or third eye chakra can inhibit its function through energy overload. Physical issues arise as oversensitivity in the lower brain (headaches), left eye (being short-sighted), ears (hearing too much background noise), nose (sensitive to smells), and the nervous system (sensitive to touch and temperature). These people are very intuition dependent, which although is not an issue from a spiritual perspective, those in the physical will have trouble with understanding information delivered by those that overuse the spiritual or third eye chakra as there will be no physical basis (no physical evidence) to back up their claims because they just know what they know to be true! A byproduct of skewed use of this chakra is that the individual may find themselves being estranged by individuals that are immersed in their incarnation.

Skewed use of the **crown chakra** results in the individual being "in their heads" too much and detached from interacting with others. This can be seen as one who thinks too much and engages little. Physically the pineal is overworked resulting with headaches in the upper brain and long-sightedness in the right eye. Again, a byproduct of skewed use of this chakra is that the individual may find themselves being estranged by individuals that are immersed in their incarnation.

## Overprotection of a Chakra or Chakra Set

What is this, I hear you exclaim, we can overprotect our chakras? Yes, we can, and this can be detrimental to the effectivity of their functionality.

We generally protect our chakras on a subconscious basis, although we can also enlist the help of a competent healer to provide appropriate protection. Appropriate protection is giving the chakra enough help in battling personal energetic attack from adverse individuals around us or from astral entities. Appropriate protection therefore gives the chakra enough protection from adversarial individuals or entities while allowing the correct and proper functionality of the chakra to continue in an unhindered way, thereby perpetuating a balanced energy system on all seven frequency levels, the gross physical and spirituo-physical.

Overprotection is when the protection is placed in a subconscious way over, in, or around the chakra as a function of total protection. Total protection effectively cuts off the chakra from the energy/ies that it is designed to work with, meaning that those energies that are needed to continue to support the energetic template that it is associated with are reduced to almost zero. The chakra, noting that it is not gaining the energy/ies to sustain the energetic template that it is associated with, works hard to pull in energy to support its role, which results in the chakra, some or all of its vortices, becoming enlarged as it fights to work with the protection in place.

Overprotection makes the chakra overwork and an overworked chakra, like everything else, can start to fail or burn out. I have seen many versions of chakra damage over the years from very minor to almost being nuked! Such is the way we treat them. Overprotection can therefore create both minor and major damage.

The ultimate issue surrounding an overprotected chakra is that it can fail, at worst generating the demise of the incarnate human vehicle, or at best, if it still has some functionality, results in energetic imbalance and physical dysfunction causing illness. I note here that most diseases caused by chakra damage manifest at the DNA level, creating diseases such as cancer, Parkinson's or Alzheimer's disease, or other rare genetic problems.

I have experienced a number of ways in which a chakra can be protected. They range from the strange to the totally practical. A few examples of what I have personally seen/experienced are described below:

1. A haze of light in front of the chakra that could resemble an energy shield.
2. A haze of light all around the chakra that could resemble an energy shield.
3. The chakra covered in an energetic version of cling film.
4. The chakra covered in a version of a hat box.
5. The chakra covered in a metal case with a padlock or other lock.
6. The chakra covered in a wooden box reinforced with steel. This looked a little like a medieval storage box or trunk.
7. An energy shield that looks like the outside has a mirrored surface.
8. The chakra covered in a bag that has a lot of spikes. This made the chakra look like a hedgehog!
9. A chakra with the open face sealed up by its own outer surface. This one looked similar to a juvenile chakra for a young incarnate.
10. A chakra that was invisible to my perception.
11. A chakra that had a filter over its face.
12. A chakra that had a mesh or gauze over its face.

These are just examples of what can be perceived by a healer when looking at a protected chakra. I am sure that other healers have not only experienced similar protection to those described above but other variations as well.

## Atrophied Chakras

A chakra can atrophy for a number of different reasons. The more prevalent reasons are attributed to skewed use or overprotection. Although a chakra that is overprotected can enlarge to compensate for the inability to draw energy of a certain frequency into it, enlargement is not the only route an overprotected chakra can take. One of the reactions of an overprotected chakra is to shut down its functionality through lack of energy flow.

The chakras themselves need energy flow to perpetuate their own existence. If the psycho-spiritual response of the incarnate Aspect or Soul is one where it desires to totally shut out the psycho-spiritually oriented emotional responses associated with that chakra, then that chakra will no longer work on maintaining its functionality and support for the energy template it is associated with.

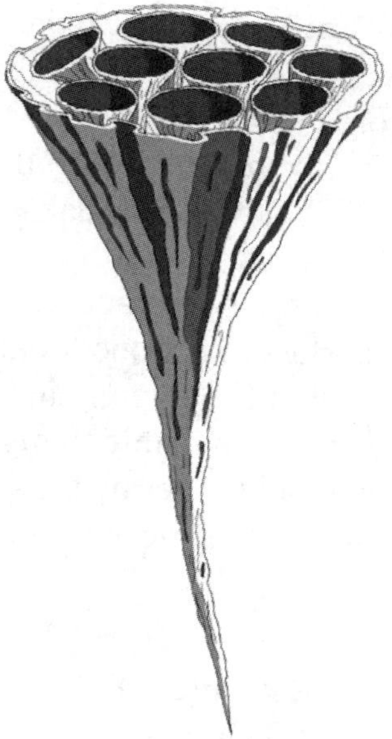

Illustration of an Atrophied Chakra

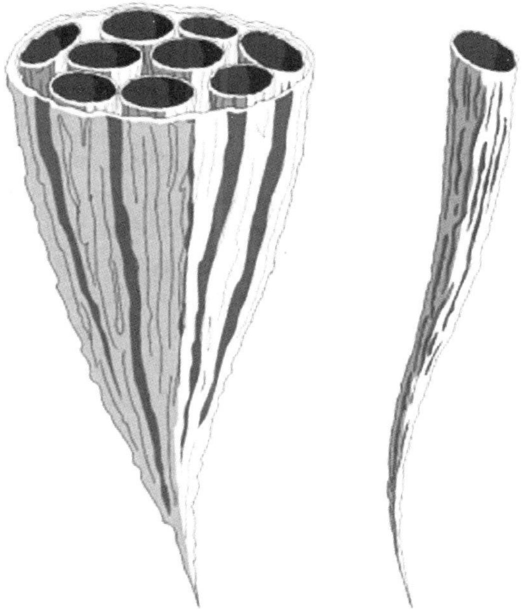

Illustration of an Atrophied Chakra with a Vortex Removed

## Foreign Objects

It is not uncommon for the healer to perceive foreign objects lodged either in between the vortices of the chakra or actually in one of the vortices.

These objects can be the product of the visual manifestation of an energetic attack by an adversarial individual, or they can be the product of what an Aspect or Soul brings with them from one incarnation to another. More often than not, the foreign object is the subconscious representation of how one of the previous incarnations was terminated, such as through war or accident. If the means of demise via foreign object was traumatic, the subconscious memory, still being fresh, brings in the energy of the method of demise and places it within the energy field, energy templates, or chakra that is within the location of the damage received by the incarnate human vehicle in that incarnation causing the chakra to operate ineffectively.

## In General

One of the things I need to point out here is that, in general, the chakras are quite hardy (robust) energetic components and that they are able to work irrespective of the vast number of detrimental ways in which we treat them. Based upon this, even though they may need healing, the very fact that one is still incarnate means that they are working at a level that can sustain one's incarnation. Sometimes this is only just about enough. If they did not function at even a minimal level, one's incarnate vehicle would demise and one would be back in the energetic. Therefore, one's physical appearance and health can be, and is, an accurate indicator of the condition of our chakras.

# Chakra Repair and Reconstruction

## A word of advice

Before I go any further, one needs to understand that working on a chakra is a very serious matter. The healer needs to receive close and in-depth instruction and guidance from a very competent healer and teacher before even considering working on any aspect of chakra repair or reconstruction on their own.

I also want to bring to the attention of the reader that the healer cannot just go ahead and work on a chakra per se. The healer needs to raise the frequencies of their own energies to that of the chakra that they need to work on.

Although the chakras are a pan-frequential energetic component and are perceivable across all of the gross physical and spirituo-physical frequencies of the incarnate human vehicle (frequency levels 1 through 7), each of the chakras are predominantly represented on and by the frequency they are designed to function with. As a result, the healer can only affect a healing on, for example, the front aspect of the solar chakra, the third chakra, when the healer is working on the third frequency level. The front aspect of the solar chakra, the third chakra, cannot be healed on the first, second, fourth, fifth, sixth, or seventh frequencies.

For example, to work on the base or root chakra, the healer needs to raise their own frequency to that of the base or root chakra, which is the first frequency. To work on the heart chakra, the healer needs to raise their own frequency to that of the heart chakra, which is the fourth frequency. And to work on the crown chakra, the healer needs to raise their own frequency to that of the crown chakra, which is the seventh frequency.

## How to Raise One's Frequencies to that of the Chakra to be Healed

Below is an exercise to help the healer raise their own frequency to that of the chakra that needs healing. Please note that this is a cumulative effect and one cannot move to the fourth frequency level by just opening the heart chakra, one also needs to open the base or root chakra, the sacral chakra, and the solar chakra before opening the heart chakra.

The location of origin of each of the chakras is as follows (from a vertical perspective):

1. The first chakra, the base or root chakra, has its point of origin in the groin, where the two legs meet the lower body.
2. The second chakra, the sacral chakra, has its point of origin 3 inches (7.5 cm) below the navel.
3. The third chakra, the solar chakra, has its point of origin 3 inches (7.5 cm) above the navel.
4. The fourth chakra, the heart chakra, has its point of origin in the sternum, at the center of the front of the chest.
5. The fifth chakra, the throat chakra, has its point of origin at the center of the front of the neck.
6. The sixth chakra, the spiritual or third eye chakra, has its point of origin at the center of the forehead, in between the eyebrows and above the bridge of the nose. (Note that the

sixth or spiritual/third eye chakra is NOT the spiritual or third eye.)

7. The seventh chakra, the crown chakra, has its point of origin at the center of the top of the head.

Be aware that there is only one of each of the vertically opposed chakras, the base or root chakra and the crown chakra. There are two of each of the horizontally opposed chakras, the sacral, solar, heart, throat, and spiritual or third eye chakras.

With the horizontally opposed chakras there are psycho-spiritual functions to consider. The front chakras are our intention, the rear chakras are our actions. As a result, anything that affects the front chakras also automatically affects the rear chakra. When one wants to open the front aspect of the fifth or throat chakra, the rear aspect of the fifth or throat chakra automatically opens. It is because of this that when we raise our frequencies to work on any of the chakras, we only need to consider the front chakras when opening the chakras to raise our frequency and can ignore the rear aspects. This does not mean that we can ignore healing the rear aspects of one of the horizontally opposed chakras for they can demand different healing requirements from those of the front aspects.

The chakra opening exercise below therefore only considers opening the front horizontally opposed chakras.

1. 1. Find a quiet room where you will not be disturbed.

2. 2. Stand with your knees slightly bent, feet shoulder width apart, arms and hands by your side. Close the eyes and focus the closed eye vision on the origin of the spiritual or third eye, which is in the same location as the spiritual or third eye chakra, BUT IS NOT

THE SPIRITUAL OR THIRD EYE itself. The location of the spiritual or third eye is at the center of the front of the forehead, in between the eyebrows and above the bridge of the nose.

If one desires to sit, one should find a straight-backed chair, place the feet flat on the ground, sit with a straight spine, place the palms of the hands uppermost upon the upper thighs. Close the eyes and focus the closed eye vision on the origin of the spiritual or third eye, which is in the same location as the spiritual or third eye chakra.

Note that the text below refers to visualization. If one has difficulty in visualizing, one can use the method of using MENTALLY SPOKEN WORDS, stating the objective quietly in the mind or under one's breath. Mentally spoken words are just as powerful as visualization because one is using one's intention to achieve the opening of a chakra (or indeed anything else). It is one's intention that counts above all else. It is the most powerful of our spiritual functions. Mentally spoken word examples are as follows:

## To Open a Chakra

*I extend my (for example) second chakra, my sacral chakra, to its maximum extension of 12 inches (or 30 cm) from its point of origin and rotate it clockwise.* The chakra will follow this intention and will extend and rotate.

## To Close a Chakra

*I stop the rotation of my (for example) second chakra, and contract it back to its point of origin.* The chakra will follow this intention and will stop rotating and contract back to its point of origin.

In most cases the healer will feel physical feedback (sensations) when on different frequency levels. Try to make a note of them when prompted below.

1. Each chakra is associated with an energetic template on a frequency level and subsequent auric level. Imagine them opening in order. This will allow you to ascend to the frequency required to heal the chakra you need to work on.

2. Concentrate on your base chakra. Imagine it (or use your mentally spoken word to achieve the same thing) as a cone and extend it vertically downward from its point of origin out to its full extension of 9 to 12 inches (30 cm). Then rotate it clockwise. To assist you in the correct rotation, imagine you have a clock on the floor and that your chakra rotation is mirroring the second hand rotating from left to right. When a chakra is fully extended and rotated in this way it effectively opens it, allowing it to receive the energies necessary to invoke the first energetic template frequency and the first Auric layer—the etheric—allowing you to also assume this level. Feel the energies that being on this level, the etheric level, Level 1 gives you. Do you feel tingling, see colors or images in your closed-eye vision, feel heat/cold, feel pressures around your head, experience emotional changes? These are all signs that your physical body is experiencing the energies associated with this level; they are proof of this change in frequency. Make a mental note of it.

3. Move on to the second chakra, the sacral. Imagine it (or use your mentally spoken word

to achieve the same thing) as a cone and extend it horizontally in front of you from its point of origin, out to its full extension of 9 to 12 inches (30 cm). Then rotate it clockwise. To assist you in the correct rotation, imagine you have a clock on a wall in front of you and that your chakra rotation is mirroring the second hand rotating from left to right. When a chakra is fully extended and rotated in this way it effectively opens it, allowing it to receive the energies necessary to invoke the second energetic template frequency and second Auric layer—the emotional layer—allowing us to also assume this level. Feel the energies of being on this level, the emotional level. Do you feel tingling, see colors or images in your closed-eye vision, feel heat/cold, feel pressures around your head, experience emotional changes? These are all signs that your physical body is experiencing the energies associated with this level; they are proof of this change in frequency. What is the change in this level compared to that experienced in the previous level? Make a mental note of it.

4. Move on to the third chakra, the solar. Imagine it (or use your mentally spoken word to achieve the same thing) as a cone and extend it horizontally in front of you, from its point of origin, out to its full extension of 9 to 12 inches (30 cm). Then rotate it clockwise. To assist you in the correct rotation, imagine you have a clock on a wall in front of you and that your chakra rotation is mirroring the second hand rotating from left to right.

When a chakra is fully extended and rotated in this way it effectively opens it, allowing it to receive the energies necessary to invoke the third energetic template frequency and third Auric layer—the mental body layer—allowing us to also assume this level. Feel the energies of being on this level, the mental body level. Do you feel tingling, see colors or images in your closed-eye vision, feel heat/cold, feel pressures around your head, experience emotional changes? These are all signs that your physical body is experiencing the energies associated with this level; they are proof of this change in frequency. What is the change in this level compared to that experienced in the previous level? Make a mental note of it.

5. Move on to the fourth chakra, the heart. Imagine it (or use your mentally spoken word to achieve the same thing) as a cone and extend it horizontally in front of you, from its point of origin out to its full extension of 9 to 12 inches (30 cm). Then rotate it clockwise. To assist you in the correct rotation, imagine you have a clock on a wall in front of you and that your chakra rotation is mirroring the second hand rotating from left to right. When a chakra is fully extended and rotated in this way it effectively opens it, allowing it to receive the energies necessary to invoke the fourth energetic template frequency and fourth Auric layer—the astral layer—allowing us to also assume this level. Feel the energies of being on this level, the astral level. Do you feel tingling, see colors

or images in your closed-eye vision, feel heat/cold, feel pressures around your head, experience emotional changes? These are all signs that your physical body is experiencing the energies associated with this level; they are proof of this change in frequency. What is the change in this level compared to that experienced in the previous level? Make a mental note of it.

6. Move on to the fifth chakra, the throat. Imagine it (or use your mentally spoken word to achieve the same thing) as a cone and extend it horizontally in front of you, from its point of origin, out to its full extension of 9 to 12 inches (30 cm). Then rotate it clockwise. To assist you in the correct rotation, imagine you have a clock on a wall in front of you and that your chakra rotation is mirroring the second hand rotating from left to right. When a chakra is fully extended and rotated in this way it effectively opens it, allowing it to receive the energies necessary to invoke the fifth energetic template frequency and fifth Auric layer—the etheric template layer—allowing us to also assume this level. Feel the energies of being on this level, the etheric template level. Do you feel tingling, are they getting finer? Do you see colors or images in your closed-eye vision, feel heat/cold, feel pressures around your head, experience emotional changes? These are all signs that your physical body is experiencing the energies associated with this level; they are proof of this change in frequency. What is the change in this level compared to that experienced in the previous

level? Make a mental note of it.

7. Move on to the sixth chakra, the third or spiritual eye. Imagine it (or use your mentally spoken word to achieve the same thing) as a cone and extend it horizontally in front of you, from its point of origin, out to its full extension of 9 to 12 inches (30 cm). Then rotate it clockwise. To assist you in the correct rotation, imagine you have a clock on a wall in front of you and that your chakra rotation is mirroring the second hand rotating from left to right. When a chakra is fully extended and rotated in this way it effectively opens it, allowing it to receive the energies necessary to invoke the sixth energetic template frequency and sixth Auric layer—the celestial body layer—allowing us to also assume this level. Feel the energies of being on this level, the celestial body level. Do you feel tingling; are they getting still finer? Do you see colors or images in your closed-eye vision, feel heat/cold, feel pressures around your head, experience emotional changes? These are all signs that your physical body is experiencing the energies associated with this level; they are proof of this change in frequency. What is the change in this level compared to that experienced in the previous level? Make a mental note of it.

8. Finally move on to the seventh chakra, the crown. Imagine it (or use your mentally spoken word to achieve the same thing) as a cone and extend it up toward the ceiling, from its point of origin, vertically out to its full extension of 9 to 12 inches (30 cm).

Then rotate it clockwise. To assist you in the correct rotation, imagine you have a clock on the ceiling above you and that your chakra rotation is mirroring the second hand rotating from left to right. When a chakra is fully extended and rotated in this way it effectively opens it allowing it to receive the energies necessary to invoke the seventh energetic template frequency and seventh Auric layer—the ketheric template layer—allowing us to also assume this level. Feel the energies of being on this level, the ketheric template level. Do you feel tingling? Are they getting still finer or have they gone? Do you see colors or images in your closed-eye vision, feel heat/cold, feel pressures around your head, experience emotional changes? These are all signs that your physical body is experiencing the energies associated with this level; they are proof of this change in frequency. What is the change in this level compared to that experienced in the previous level? Make a mental note of it.

9. You are now at the end of the gross physicality/spirituo-physicality of your human form. Stay at this level of a few moments and absorb how you feel, what your physical body has experienced, giving you proof, physical proof, that you have actually risen above those frequencies that you are normally associated with on the Earth level, the zero level.

10. Slowly close each chakra one by one, starting at the crown chakra and finishing with the base or root chakra by first stopping the rotation of the chakra and then withdrawing

it back into its location of origin. Make a note of the feelings, the tingling sensations; are they getting coarser as you descend the frequencies? Do you see colors or images in your closed-eye vision, feel heat/cold, feel pressures around your head, experience emotional changes? The experiences, the responses that the human form gives you, should be repeated on each of the levels in the descent in reverse order of that which you experienced them on the ascent.

11. To move down from the seventh frequency level to the sixth frequency level, visualize or use your mentally spoken word to achieve the same thing, that you stop the rotation of the crown chakra and withdraw it back into the crown area of the head, its point of origin. You are now on the sixth frequency level.

12. To move down from the sixth frequency level to the fifth frequency level, visualize or use your mentally spoken word to achieve the same thing, that you stop the rotation of the spiritual or third eye chakra and withdraw it back into the area in between the eyebrows and above the bridge of the nose, its point of origin. You are now on the fifth frequency level.

13. To move down from the fifth frequency level to the fourth frequency level, visualize or use your mentally spoken word to achieve the same thing, that you stop the rotation of the throat chakra and withdraw it back into the center of the front of the throat, its point of origin. You are now on the fourth frequency

level.

14. To move down from the fourth frequency level to the third frequency level, visualize or use your mentally spoken word to achieve the same thing, that you stop the rotation of the heart chakra and withdraw it back into the area in the center of the front of the chest, the sternum, its point of origin. You are now on the third frequency level.

15. To move down from the third frequency level to the second frequency level, visualize or use your mentally spoken word to achieve the same thing, that you stop the rotation of the solar chakra and withdraw it back into the area 3 inches (7.5 cm) above the navel, its point of origin. You are now on the second frequency level.

16. To move down from the second frequency level to the first frequency level, visualize or use your mentally spoken word to achieve the same thing, that you stop the rotation of the sacral chakra and withdraw it back into the area 3 inches (7.5 cm) below the navel, its point of origin. You are now on the first frequency level.

17. To move down from the first frequency level to the zero frequency level, the Earth level, visualize or use your mentally spoken word to achieve the same thing, that you stop the rotation of the base chakra and withdraw it back up into the area of the groin, where the two legs meet the lower body, its point of origin. You are now back on the zero frequency level, the Earth level.

If this is your first time performing this exercise, I recommend drinking some water to ground you and moving slowly as you may feel a little disoriented. This is normal and is nothing to worry about. Note that the healer should always return themselves to the frequencies that are classified as the zero or Earth level once a healing procedure has been completed. This is simply to ensure that the healer continues to be grounded at the frequencies that they are incarnate into and that they stay psycho-spiritually "present" in these frequencies.

I state again that for the healer under training this is a cumulative effect and one cannot move to the fourth frequency level by just opening the heart chakra; one also needs to open the base or root chakra, the sacral chakra, and the solar chakra before opening the heart chakra.

However, when one is experienced with many years of healing, the healer may be able to open all the chakras in one go. This can be done by using intention, or simply by using one's intention to go to a level in a way that replicates all of the cumulative chakras being opened.

# Establishing Which Chakra Needs Healing and What to Do

## Scanning the body

Before any healing is ventured upon, the healer needs to establish four basic sets of information:

1. What are the physical symptoms?
2. What are the emotional and psycho-spiritual responses/history?
3. What areas of the energy bodies of the incarnate human vehicle are affected?
4. How are they all linked?

From the perspective of the chakras, chakra dysfunction exhibits issues in all of the above areas to a lesser or greater extent. Predominately, though, and from an energetic perspective, chakra dysfunction manifests as poor energy flow on the energetic template aligned with the frequency that the chakra is associated with. In order to establish this, the healer needs to use both their analysis of the patient's physical issues and how the patient is emotionally and psycho-spiritually aligned while scanning the body to see where the associated energetic dysfunctions link in. In effect, the physical and psycho-spiritual responses help the healer focus on the area that needs healing straight away rather than having to scan the whole body on every frequency associated with an energy body and its associated chakra to see where the damage is.

In order to scan the human body from a very basic level, the healer needs to first place themselves on the first frequency level by opening the base or root chakra, which is achieved by extending and rotating it clockwise. Once on the first frequency level, the healer should close their eyes and mentally move around the body of the patient, gaining a picture of the energetic template and chakra. If that chakra and energetic template do not present any abnormalities, then the healer can move on to the next frequency level by extending and rotating the sacral chakra clockwise and again mentally moving around the body of the patient to observe the manifestation of any abnormalities. Abnormalities that are observed should be noted and the healer should move on to the next frequency level and the next scan. When all seven frequencies associated with the seven chakras and seven energetic templates have been scanned, a picture can be created of the work to be done. This picture will illustrate what abnormality is observed on what energetic template, on what frequency level, and with what chakra. Only when this picture is established can the healer embark on creating a list of work to be done in that healing session.

Taking into consideration that we are just looking at chakra dysfunction for the moment, we need to understand what work needs to be performed on what chakra. This can be the replacement or repair of the chakra or chakras concerned.

Scanning is an important part of the creation of the energetic prognosis of one's patient. It should be performed at the start of any new consultation, even if the patient is an existing client.

## Individual Vortices

When damage or dysfunction of a chakra is noted

in the scan, the healer can raise their frequency to that of the chakra by opening the necessary chakras. Note that if the damage is on the heart chakra there is no need to open the chakras above, only those below in the cumulative fashion. This is the same for all chakras.

The individual vortices of a chakra are those parts of the chakra that attract the subfrequencies within a frequency level or band. The higher the frequency a chakra has to work with, the higher the number of vortices that are within a chakra. This is because there are more subfrequencies in the higher and finer frequency levels than those of the lower frequencies.

The perceptual image of a chakra and its vortices is one of a cone-shaped energetic organ that is filled with smaller cones. It can be almost organic in nature, although I have perceived chakras as mechanical in nature as well. The smaller diameter of the cone is linked to the main arteries of the energy distribution network of the incarnate human vehicle with the larger diameter being open to the energies of the physical universe. When one observes the open end of a chakra with their perceptual vision one can see the larger diameters of the smaller cones that are the vortices. They appear to be a group of small cones wrapped together in a skin that is attached to the main energy distribution artery. The smaller diameters of the vortices appear to look like a tail or taproot of a root vegetable and blend into the connection of the smaller diameter of the chakra itself so that the vortices and the chakra have a single combined connection to the main energy distribution artery.

When the vortices that are damaged are observed by the healer the damage can be presented in many ways, some of which are relative to the healer's modality or method of visualization. They can appear to be burnt out, diseased, like a broken lightbulb, or some other mechanical or organic representation.

Irrespective of how the chakra, vortices, and damage present themselves to the healer, the process for removal and replacement is essentially the same. When the healer is at the correct frequency and is perceiving the chakra and the vortices, they should use their intention to visualize that they are able to pluck out the damaged vortex and place it in an energy recycling bin that the healer will have visualized. The energy associated with that vortex will therefore return to Source by reintegrating with the energies of the physical universe. Next, the healer should ask for help from Source, his/her Guide and Helpers, or the Guide and Helpers of the patient, to give the healer, or materialize in the hand of the healer, replacement vortices. The healer should then visualize that they are placing the replacement vortex into the gap left in the chakra by the damaged or diseased one. The healer who visualizes the more common imagery of the energetically organic chakra and vortices will observe the taproot or tail of the smaller diameter of the vortices blending into the combined chakra/vortices where they connect to the main energy distribution artery. The mechanical visualization may appear like the vortex has a bayonet or Edison screw fitment of a lightbulb or a computer peripheral interface connector. Whichever modality of visualization is employed by the healer, once the vortices are replaced, the efficiency of the chakra concerned will return to normality and the patient will notice a return to feeling "normal."

Although this appears to be a simple operation, it requires the skill of an educated, experienced, and capable healer who has confidence resulting from years of time in service as a healer—and not bravado.

It is quite common for the healer to note that more than one vortex within the chakra is damaged, diseased, or dysfunctional. If this is the case, then each of the vortices should be dealt with during the same healing appointment by repeating the method described above.

## Groups of Vortices

The individual vortices of a chakra can be and are grouped together relative to the subfrequencies that they are associated with, although this is not especially noticeable with the lower frequency chakras such as the base or root chakra and the sacral chakra. However, the sacral chakra does have grouped vortices but they are few and difficult to identify, and it is therefore more obvious from the solar chakra upward that there are vortices grouped together.

Vortices are grouped together according to subfrequency and, for want of a better term, bandwidth. The more vortices that are grouped together, the more bandwidth is available for a certain subfrequency for the chakra to process and use. Similarly, the more bandwidth that is available at a certain subfrequency, the more vortices are required to process the energy at that subfrequency. This function, obvious as it may seem, is a critical part of overall chakra functionality and moreover, efficiency. Based upon this, when a group of vortices have one or a number of vortices damaged or dysfunctional, the functions of the group of vortices in general are affected.

The healer may therefore encounter one or more vortices that need to be replaced within a group or a whole group that needs to be replaced.

When the healer needs to replace a cluster of vortices that are part of a group, they should replace them in the same method described above on a one-by-one basis. Similarly, when the healer needs to replace a number of vortices that are part of a number of groups, they should also replace them in the same method described above on a one-by-one basis. It is only when a whole group or most of the vortices within a group need to be replaced that one should consider replacing that group.

As with the chakras themselves, the perceptual appearance of a vortex can be either organic or mechanical in nature to the healer, depending upon how well they work with the imagery presented to them. The vortices within a group can appear to be burnt out, melted, withered, or simply broken as a result.

Groups of vortices are linked both together and all together with the chakra itself. In my experience, I perceive the vortices connected together on either a root-based system at the bottom of the group (garlic is a good example with its individual cloves joined at the root to create a bulb), or connected together in a subframe or carrier, which is in turn connected to a larger connection within the chakra, such as an array of bulbs. Note that groups of vortices can be clustered together or in circles of vortices that surround other circular groups or other clusters of vortices.

## Replacement of Groups of Vortices

The replacement of a group of vortices is similar in operation to replacing a single vortex with the exception that the healer is working with a group. Using the method described to replace a single vortex, the healer should be aware that the chakra itself needs to be treated with care at the same time.

Remember, replacing one vortex affects the function and efficiency of a chakra in a relatively minor, while still being important, way because it doesn't affect the whole receptive bandwidth. Whereas replacing a group of vortices effectively stops the chakra's functional ability to receive the whole subfrequency and its associated bandwidth. Based upon this, replacing a group of, or groups of vortices should have the same level of skill, care, and respect as a full chakra replacement with the healer.

Once establishing, via a scan, that a chakra of a certain frequency needs a group of vortices to be replaced, the healer should place themselves on the frequency of the chakra concerned and visualize the group or groups to be removed and replaced.

Work one group at a time. DO NOT REMOVE AND REPLACE ALL GROUPS TOGETHER. Visualize plucking the group, in either its organic or mechanical representation, gently by using both of your "energetic" hands. Tease the group out.

With the organic representation, the group's roots will appear to untangle slowly, disassociating from the collective of roots of the remaining groups and single "central" vortex attached to the main body of the chakra. Work the group out slowly until it is completely separated from the chakra. Next, place the old group of vortices into an energetic recycling bin that you can manifest close to you. I manifest an energetic recycling bin to my right-hand side usually. Then, as with the single vortex, visualize, or ask any entities that are helping you with the healing, to create a new group of vortices. When manifest, gently place the group back into the location where the original damaged group was positioned. You will perceive that the roots of the group in the organic representation intertwine with the roots of the existing groups and the main body of the chakra itself. Once the group has been replaced, the chakra will start to perform correctly and the healer will notice a distinct change in the energy of the main chakra. In the event that a number of groups need to be replaced, the change in the energy of the chakra may not be so discernable at first but will increase as the remaining groups are replaced, increasing one by one.

If the healer perceives the groups in a mechanical way, the group of vortices may appear to be like a group or array of bulbs, for instance, attached together on a subframe or carrier. When perceived in this way, the healer may visualize removing the damaged group by "unplugging" the group from the main chakra. Dispose of this group and manifest a new group of vortices in the same way as the organic version. The replacements can simply be "plugged in" to the same location as the old damaged group. As with the organic version, the change in energy of the chakra can be perceived by the healer, either by a marked change if only one group is needed to be replaced or in slight stepped changes if a number of groups need to be replaced.

Whichever method of visualization is perceived, not only will a change in energy be detected by the healer energetically, but it will also be detected by the patient in terms of how they feel. The physical appearance of the patient also changes to suit the renewed functionality and efficiency of the overall chakra and can be easily observed by anyone in the same space as the healer and the patient.

## Outer Skin

Every chakra is the collective product of its vortices grouped together either individually, in clustered groups or circles of groups, and then surrounded by an outer skin to create the overall appearance of a chakra. This outer skin or covering is used to keep the vortices in one location and not allow them to spread or move around their area of connectivity with the rest of the energy network associated with the frequencies that they are designed to work with and those of the other frequencies that create the incarnate human vehicle. This skin also protects the vortices. In the event that this outer skin is damaged in any way, it is possible that a vortex or small group or cluster of vortices can protrude out of the boundary that the outer skin produces. When a vortex or group of vortices is/are outside of this skin, the overall balance of the functionality of the chakra is adversely affected creating energetic and spirituo-physical dysfunction.

Any damage to a chakra or its vortices results in the patient feeling discomfort in the area of origin of the affected chakra and even lack of stability or energy. Damage to the outer skin or covering of a chakra also produces these symptoms. It can be classified as a "hernia" of the chakra and needs to be dealt with on an urgent basis.

There are two main ways in which the outer skin of a chakra can be healed or repaired. The first way is to actually repair the area of damage or tear; the second way is to replace the outer skin in totality.

## Repairing the Outer Skin

A damaged outer skin results in the energies and frequencies associated with the chakra being healed to appear to leak out of the area of damage.

When repairing the outer skin of a chakra, the healer

should open the chakras required to place the healer at the frequency associated with the chakra to be healed. The area of damage or tear will be visualized by the healer as either a tear or rip in fabric of some sort relative to how the healer visualizes wounds or as an organic representation such as a burn, contusion, incision, or avulsion (tear) of the skin away from the chakra.

In both instances, the healer should visualize the outer skin being repaired by either "darning" the material type presented to them or by visualizing the skin healing, in a similar way to how the physical skin heals but in a greatly accelerated way. The healer can also create a 3D matrix around the area to be healed, bridging the gap between the areas of good outer skin and the void or damaged area. Visualize this matrix being slowly filled up with energy, the energy recreating the area of outer skin that needs to be repaired or replaced.

Once you have decided on the type of visualization you are perceiving and the method to use to heal the damage to the chakra's outer skin, and the healing has been completed, the outer skin of the chakra should be consistent in its presentation all around the chakra, illustrating a healthy outer skin and fully protected vortices.

## Replacing the Outer Skin

Again, if damaged, the energies and frequencies associated with the chakra being healed may appear to leak out of the area of damage. In the event that the outer skin has, in the opinion of the healer, too much damage to warrant a repair, the whole outer skin can be replaced.

As with other work on the chakras and/or vortices, when replacing the outer skin of a chakra, the healer should open the chakras required to place the healer at the frequency associated with the chakra to be healed.

Once at the correct frequency, the healer should visualize the outer skin of the chakra in the way that they best perceive the chakra and its outer skin. The outer skin can be represented as fabric, skin, or a plastic cover. To replace the skin in whatever representation perceived, the healer should visualize that they slowly peel the outer skin from around the vortices, the vortices being perceived as being held all together in fresh air, so to speak. With the outer configuration of the vortices exposed but protecting the inner configurations of vortices, the outer skin should be disposed of by using the recycling bin as previously described, allowing the energy to be returned back to Source. The healer can then manifest a new outer skin by using their intention or by asking their Guide and Helpers, the patient's Guide and Helpers or any trusted entity that they work with that assists them with their healing work. Once the new outer skin is manifest or materialized into the energetic hand of the healer, they should visualize reintroducing/recovering the vortices that form the outer configuration. Once the new skin has been reintroduced, the chakra will appear normal and the energies at the frequency associated with that chakra will no longer leak out of the outer skin.

## Chakra Replacement

The replacement of a chakra is a very serious procedure, even if it appears to be simple, and the healer who embarks upon such a healing needs to have received comprehensive instruction from a competent teacher, who will have observed the healer during the first few chakra replacement procedures. Considerable practice is suggested before "going solo" and performing a chakra replacement on one's own without the backup of one's teacher.

Remember when replacing a chakra, the patient will spend a short period of time actually without that chakra so the healer may ask The Source to sustain the patient with the energies at the frequencies received by the chakra concerned, or use their own energy to do the same. However, appropriating energy from The Source is the most preferable solution to this problem and should always be the primary route for the healer.

All this being said, the replacement of a chakra is very similar to the replacement of an individual vortex. The healer should raise their frequency to that of the chakra being replaced and visualize the chakra to be replaced in the way that they are comfortable with. As with the vortices, the chakra can appear to be either organic or mechanical in representation. The damage to the chakra may present itself as either being burnt out, withered, or simply damaged by what would appear to be from an impact of some sort.

## Removal of Astral Entities Linked into a Chakra

Astral entities exist in the frequencies associated with the fourth, fifth, sixth, and seventh frequencies of our universal environment. The fourth is the lower astral; the fifth, the upper lower astral; the sixth, the lower upper astral; and the seventh, the upper astral. Their existence is transitory because they cannot maintain their own existence through the metabolization of their own energy and therefore, they take energy from other, higher and usually incarnate, entities.

They are created in two ways, either by us as human beings as a function of desire, or personal energetic attack, or adversarial thoughts aimed toward another, or by the normal evolution of energy coalescing together (see *The Origin Speaks* for a detailed explanation of how an energy can become sentient —*GSN*). Astral entities, however, only have a level of intelligence that revolves around their survival or perpetuated existence through the appropriation of energy from those entities or beings that are incarnate. Some of this intelligence is detailed enough to allow the astral entity to create a symbiotic relationship with an incarnate host by making them feel powerful or by controlling the host in some way.

There are many ways in which an astral entity attaches itself to a host and we will deal with others later in this book. However, it is through direct connection to a chakra that the astral entity prefers to employ because the chakra is an energy receiver for the host and therefore delivers pure, high-quality energetic sustenance.

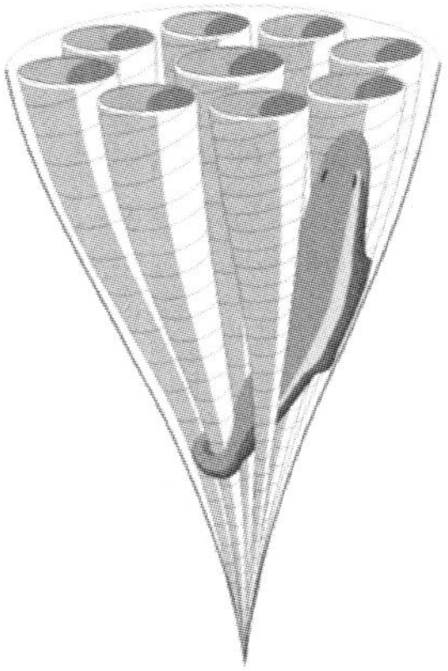

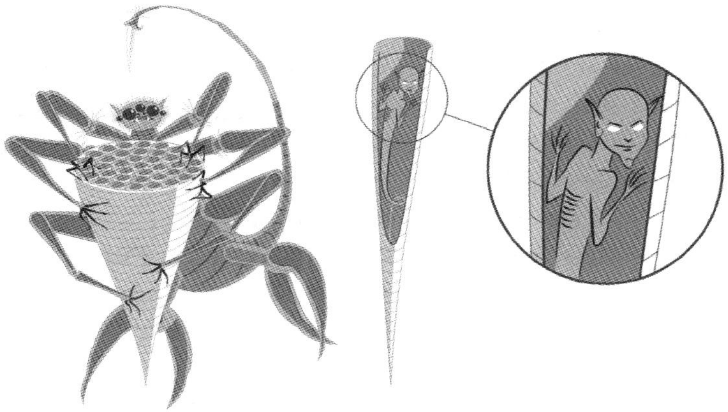

In most cases therefore, the person will become the host either as a result of the astral entity being the subject of the astral entity's creation, and use, as an attacking or adversarial medium, or through it being drawn to the potential host in its need to gain energy to perpetuate its existence.

When removing an astral entity from a chakra, the healer first needs to establish if an astral entity is the predominant reason for chakra dysfunction by the use of the full body, and therefore chakra scan previously described. Once the dysfunction of a chakra is identified as a function of astral entity attachment, the healer then needs to check that the astral entity is only associated with the frequency that the chakra of interest is associated with. When an astral entity is attached to any other part of the incarnate human vehicle other than a chakra, it can be manifest on any or all of the gross physical and spirituo-physical frequencies and as a result, the removal of that entity must be performed on some or all seven gross physical and spirituo-physical frequencies. However, it is normal for an astral entity to be predominantly associated with the frequencies of the chakra that it is attached to, and not detected on the other frequency levels. If this is the case, then the astral entity only needs to be removed from the frequency of the chakra that it is attached to and no other.

I do note here that although an astral entity may choose attachment to any of the chakras associated with the incarnate human form, when they are manifest to perform some sort of adversarial or attacking response, they are usually found in and around the heart chakra, the fourth frequency level.

Once the healer has established what chakra the astral entity is taking energy from, the healer must open their own chakra/s to elevate themselves to the frequency of the chakra that the entity is going to be removed from.

The astral entity will undoubtedly try to defend itself and may present a shape or form to the healer that they find abhorrent or are fearful of. If this is the case, the healer must be aware that they are significantly more powerful than the astral entity and should not pay any attention to how big or fearful the image presented to the healer is. Any fear projected from the healer will be used against the healer by the astral entity and be projected back to them. The healer will then, in most cases, consider that the job of removing the entity is too big or too difficult for them and will abandon the healing work.

A competent and well-trained healer will ignore any

defensive responses by the astral entity and continue with the task of removal. Please be aware that removing an astral entity from a chakra is delicate work and care must be taken to not damage the chakra as a result of removing the entity from the chakra.

Once at the correct frequency, and observing the astral entity with their perception, the healer can then visualize removing the entity by taking full grip of the entity with both energetic hands. Gently and firmly take hold of the entity in the same way as you might a wriggling cat from a friend or partner's lap, safely extracting the cat's claws from their clothing. As with the wriggling cat example, the astral entity may decide to "hang on" to the chakra so be prepared to move the entity around in a few angles of movement or employ a "third" energetic arm and hand or even enlist the help of a trusted entity that helps with healing such as a healing entity or your Guide or one of its Helpers to lend another hand. Again be careful not to cause damage to the vortices or external skin or covering of the chakra by removing the astral entity. When you have teased the astral entity away from the chakra, the healer can send the entity back to the light, so to speak, so that its energy can be recycled by The Source by the use of visualizing the recycling bin as previously described and placing the entity within it.

In the event that the chakra sustained some damage as a result of removing the astral entity, the affected vortices, or outer skin, or cover of the chakra can be healed by using the techniques previously described.

I stated that in most cases an astral entity that is attached to a chakra is usually predominantly represented on the frequency of the chakra the entity is taking energy from. If this is not the case, then the healer will need to establish, via scanning the patient, which of the remaining chakras are also affected and repeat this work on each of them one by one, including any potential repair work created by removing the entity from the chakra.

It is also worth noting that if an astral entity is attached to more than one chakra that the healer is advised to work on removing the entity from the lowest frequency chakra, performing any repair work first, before moving on to the next highest frequency chakra. As the healer moves up the frequencies, they will notice that the work of removing the astral entity from the chakra and performing any repair work becomes faster and faster the higher up the frequencies they work.

Removal of an astral entity from the chakra of a patient usually results in an immediate and positive response. If, however, this is not the case then the healer needs to revisit the need to scan the patient's energetic bodies to look for other, smaller entities that may have been missed and remove them as well.

I will discuss the removal of an astral entity from other areas of the incarnate human vehicle in a chapter devoted to this subject.

## Removal of Foreign Objects in a Chakra

It is not uncommon to have the energetic representation of a past life or current life trauma that has affected the incarnate Aspect at the very core of its being. The trauma being at a fundamental level that is both physical and emotional/psychological and lodged within a chakra. The representation can be illustrated as a way or method in which the Aspect previously left its last or other incarnations.

Those Aspects that left their last incarnation as a function of conflict or a battle within a war may have the energy associated with their incarnate vehicles' death represented by the means in which they demised, such as by spear, sword, knife, bullet, shrapnel, or blunt instrument interrupting the function of a chakra.

Those Aspects that left their last incarnation as a function of accident may have the energy associated with their incarnate vehicles' death represented by the means in which they demised, such as by being crushed by a vehicle or debris, impaled by debris, limbs severed, explosion, poisoned, gassed, falling, drowning, or burnt.

The energy associated with an accident can be expressed in any part of the gross physical and spirituo-physical aspect of the incarnate human vehicle and not specifically a chakra. Based upon this, I will only discuss the removal of debris from a chakra as a result of accident as this is identical to the demise of the incarnate human vehicle as a function of conflict illustrated above. The remaining detail is identical to that of the demise of the incarnate human vehicle in past lives not associated with a weapon or debris specifically interrupting the function of a chakra and will be discussed within its own chapter.

When a chakra has a foreign object, of any of those described above, lodged within it its function is impaired and the energy accrued by it is interrupted causing an energy imbalance that affects the function of the energetic template that is predominantly represented by the chakra concerned. The gross physical organs anatomically associated with that chakra are also therefore affected, creating health issues on the gross physical levels and, depending upon the resolve of the incarnate Aspect, the psycho-spiritual functions associated with that chakra are also affected creating emotional and psychological issues.

## Establishing the Need for Removing a Foreign Object from a Chakra

To remove a foreign object from a chakra, the healer must have first established that there is an issue with the functionality of one of the patient's chakras that requires detailed analysis. This can be achieved by normal scanning of the patient's body, energy system, and chakras. Secondly, that the detailed analysis is performed one frequency at a time, by the healer opening their chakras one chakra at a time, so that each of the chakras can be observed and analyzed. This is to ensure that only the chakra or chakras that need to be worked on are in fact worked on, that the energetic representation of the foreign object is recognized, and the scope of the work needed to remove it is established. Additionally, the healer will also be able to establish whether any links to a past life or indeed past lives need to be severed as part of the healing process.

Once all of the above has been established the healer can commence the task of removing the foreign object from the chakra. Although any past life associations can also be actioned once the foreign object is removed, the detail behind such healing will be discussed in a chapter dedicated to this subject.

To remove the foreign object from the chakra, the healer must elevate their frequency to that of the chakra concerned by opening their own chakra/s one by one until the healer is at the same frequency as that of the chakra of concern. This process gets quicker the more competent the healer becomes.

Using visualization (clairvoyance), the healer should observe how the foreign object is attached or lodged within the structure of the chakra and if it is also affecting the energetic template associated with that chakra. If the foreign object is only lodged within the chakra, then the healer will only need to work on removing the object from the chakra. If, however, the object is also interfering with (impaled within) the energetic template associated with the chakra, then the healer will need to ensure that they also remove the object from the energetic template at the same time as removing it from the chakra. Not removing the foreign object from the energetic template at the same time as the chakra can result in the energy associated with the foreign object still causing an issue with the energetic template and the chakra as by previous association.

For the benefit of efficiency, I will describe the process of removing the foreign object from both the chakra and the energetic template.

Once the healer has elevated to the correct frequency level and has visualized the energy affecting the chakra and energy template in the way it has presented itself to the healer as a foreign object in one of the ways previously described, the healer can establish how best to remove that object.

The healer should work on removing the foreign object as if it was solid, visualizing using the hands to gently move the object out of the energetic template and the chakra. The chakra and the energy template should be treated with the same care as a consultant surgeon would treat a major organ, ensuring that they don't create more damage in removing the object than has already been caused by it. If need be, the healer should twist and turn the object to avoid tearing any of the small 3D energy lines or grids that represent the energy template on the level he/she is working on. For example, I have seen foreign objects that have barbs like fishhooks which can tear the energy lines of the energy template. The energy vortices can be moved to one side, or if damaged, removed from the chakra at the same time as the object is being removed from the chakra. The object can also be twisted and turned to avoid other healthy vortices within the chakra. Do not try to break the foreign object to assist in its removal as this will allow some of the energies associated with it to disperse around the energy template and chakra of the patient, which will need to be cleaned and cleared. It cannot be left within the energies of the patient because it will create residual issues associated with the foreign object. Once the object has been removed, it can be discarded into a recycling bin that the healer can manifest close by, using their intention to make anything that is placed within it get sent back to The Source.

Once the object has been removed, the healer needs to clean the damaged areas energetically. This can be done by the healer visualizing the damaged area being surrounded or bathed in silver light. In the gross physical, silver has antibacterial and antimicrobial properties. In the metaphysical, it has the ability to act as a sterilizing agent and actively promote healing. I use it to cleanse and sterilize the damaged areas of all aspects of the incarnate human vehicle.

Once cleansed, the energetic template can be repaired by considering it as a 3D grid or net, the damaged areas being represented by tears in the 3D grid or net. To repair this 3D grid or net, the healer should visualize reconnecting the tears with the undamaged aspects of the grid or net. One example of how to reconnect the tears is to visualize stitching or darning the damaged area to the good area in a similar way that one would darn or repair an item of clothing. The healer will observe a change in the appearance of the energetic template when the 3D grid or net is repaired. I usually see the template glow iridescently. The damaged aspects of the chakra, such as the outer covering or skin and the vortices, can be repaired or replaced in the ways described in the sections above.

## Removal of Protection

### The Two Types of Protection

When I talk about the need for the removal of protection from a chakra I can imagine that this section will raise a few eyebrows among the healing fraternity. However, there are two types of protection generated by the patient and this is why we need to consider the actual need for the removal of chakra protection rather than leaving it in place. The first method of protection is one that is generated by the incarnate Aspect (Soul) as an automatic function of protection from adversarial contact with another and is all encompassing to the point of overprotection. The second method of protection is a function of the mindful application of protection and is designed to provide specific protection only.

I will elaborate further on the two versions, I may repeat myself.

With the first method of chakra protection, we automatically protect our chakras when we encounter adversarial people or environments that we meet in our daily lives. Because the protection is automatic there are no graduations in the level of protection generated, or indeed how and when to remove this protection. It is usually a function of the "fight or flight" response and is created in a spontaneous manner. When this type of protection is created, it is "total" in its application. By total I mean that it is designed to stop any form of energetic interaction with the chakra. Total protection, however, also results in the interference of the chakra's ability to pull in energy to support the energetic template that it is associated with and ultimately affects the physical health of the incarnate human vehicle.

The visual representation of this type of protection depends upon the personality of the incarnate Aspect and can range from what appears to be similar to cling film, to hardened steel boxes that are welded together to cast-iron boxes that look like a money safe complete with combination lock to wooden medieval doors to dense bramble bushes complete with thorns. All of these illustrations indicate a state of "don't come near me" energetically, which makes it difficult for the healer to help the patient by removing the protection, restore chakra function, and provide a more appropriate level of protection.

The second type of protection is usually generated by an incarnate Aspect that is of a higher frequency. This person will be more intuitive and more aware and awake and as a result will know when they need to create protection for their chakra/s, and at what level or focus, depending on whether it is for the interaction with an adversarial individual, environment, or both. They will also know if they need to have several different levels and types of protection to cope with various different individuals or environments and will actively and consciously swap between levels and types of protection. More importantly, they will know that they need to protect the chakra "while" allowing it to function properly. This allows the chakra to "pull in" or "accept" essential energy to perpetuate the incarnate Aspect's ability to animate the incarnate human vehicle at the frequency level of that chakra while being appropriately protected.

When I look at the visualizations of the types and levels of protection of an aware and awake individual, I see versions of those visualizations described above but they appear to be subtler in their application. By that, I mean they have what I can only describe as a transparent appearance to them when one looks directly at them. When the creator wants the chakra to function correctly and pull in or receive energy, the protection becomes more transparent. When the creator thinks about an adversarial individual, the protection becomes solid in appearance. It is quite normal for this type of protection to have the appearance of a two-way mirror or an energy field surrounding the chakra concerned.

When considering that the healer may need to remove any protection from a chakra, one first needs to understand if the patient is on a high/er frequency and is more aware and awake, because if they are, then they will be actively "modulating" the level and type of protection around the chakra to suit their needs. If this is the case, then there is no need for the healer to remove any protection because it is under conscious control. Therefore, the second version of protection does not normally need to be removed and we can concentrate on the first version in isolation.

## Illustrations of Types of Protection

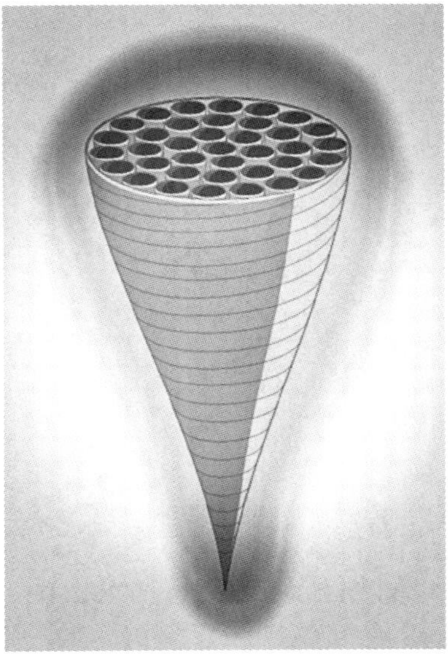

A Haze of Energy Surrounding a Chakra

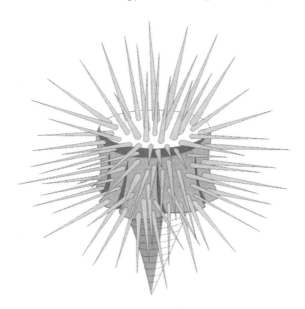

A Chakra Covered in a Bag Full of Spikes as Protection

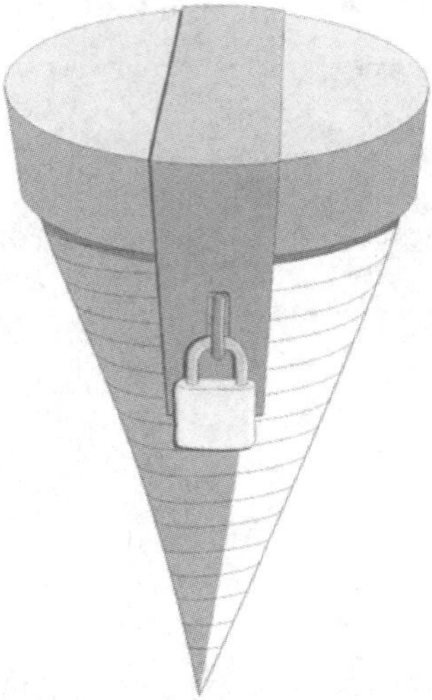

A Hat Box Type of Protection

## Removing the Old Protection, Replacing with Appropriate Protection

As with all healing described in this book, the healer first needs to elevate their own frequency to the frequency level of the chakra whose protection needs to be removed and replaced. This can be achieved by the healer opening their own chakras using the methods previously described. Also, the healer needs to obtain the permission of the patient to remove and replace the protection. This is a fundamental request in any healing modality and is not just relative to working on the chakras and their protection.

When at the correct frequency level and observing the visualization of the protection with the mind's eye, the healer should create a strategy of how to safely and carefully remove the protection without damaging the chakra or its vortices. This strategy should involve the creation of the "tools" necessary to open, unlock, cut open, disassemble, and remove the protection in the way one would if working with actual physical protection of the sort visualized. I have observed the need to create energy that resembles such tools as drills, lasers, lock picks, wood saws, hack (metal) saws, chisels (both wood and metal), screwdrivers, and grinders, such is the level of protection created and the subsequent resistance experienced by high levels of total protection!

Once the healer has established a strategy and has created or visualized the tools to action the strategy, the healer can then slowly and methodically start the task of opening or dismantling the protection. The healer can ask for the help of an entity that is committed to be of service via healing or even ask for help from their Guide and Helpers, the Guide and Helpers of the patient, or even The Source.

To help the reader, I feel it will be useful to describe a process I used to remove a very thorough type and level of protection.

One of the types and levels of protection I have worked on was a hardened steel box (previously mentioned) that was encasing the solar chakra of a patient.

When observing this type of protection, the healer should note whether or not the hardened steel box has the appearance of being welded or riveted together. This will suggest which method of dismantling the protection should be employed. Rivets can be both drilled out and ground off using the visualization of the energy associated with such physical tools as a hand drill or an angle grinder. Establish where the best point to start is, such as the natural weak point offered by a door, or if no door is presented to the healer, the place that allows the easiest method of starting the disassembly.

Again, the healer should visualize a recycling bin where the components of the protection can be placed and the energy associated with them can be recycled by The Source.

If rivets are observed, visualize a portable hand drill with the correct size drill bit or an angle grinder with a "metal-cutting" wheel. Gently grind or drill off the rivet heads that can be observed from the panel that has been chosen to be removed first. If welding is observed, use the same angle grinder visualization to gradually remove the welds that you can see. In either case, detach the first panel that you have chosen by removing all of the rivets or welds until the panel feels like it should fall off. Remove the panel carefully and then move to the other sides or panels.

I expect there to be six panels or sides, a top, four sides, and one base that would be protecting the area of the chakra where it enters the energy template associated with it and attaches to the main energy distribution network (artery) that connects all of the main chakras together. The sides will be easier to remove than the top and will be removed using the same or similar method and "tools." Once the healer has removed the first five sides or panels, the healer is faced with the hardest task when removing chakra protection because the last panel may well be integrated with the energy template that the chakra is associated with. If it is, the healer will need to treat the area that it is integrated with in the same way as removing the energy associated with a weapon or debris lodged in a chakra or associated energy template as described previously. Undoubtedly, the healer will need to remove the final panel by cutting it from two ends that are diametrically opposed to each other. In this example, this can be achieved by using the energies associated with the angle grinding tool splitting the final panel into two pieces being careful NOT TO TOUCH the chakra or its associated energy template with the visualized angle grinder because this will damage the chakra and/or the energy template.

Once the final panel or side is in two pieces, carefully remove it and place it in your recycling bin. If it is integrated into the energy template, gradually tease it out and away from the energies associated with the energy template concerned. Once the protection is removed, bathe the chakra and the local area of the energy template in silver light to assist in any need for healing.

In the event that further protection of the chakra or chakras is required by the patient, then the healer can guide the patient in applying chakra protection of the second version by asking them to visualize that the chakra is surrounded by a dome of energy that has the appearance and properties of a two-way mirror. This two-way mirror dome should be programmed, by using the patient's "intention," to only allow energy "IN" from the universe or Source and reject any energy that is adversarial, irrespective of where it comes from, such as a work colleague, family member, friend, or loved one. Energy "OUT" can be projected as normal to ensure that the normal modalities of communication that use the chakras or are used by the chakras are uninhibited.

Other types of protection such as medieval wooden doors or thorn bushes should be removed with care by the healer visualizing the correct tools that they would use to remove the physical representations of the visualizations of protection from a physical body, should they surround part or all of it. The total protection of a patient can be administered by the patient themselves by using a number of ways taught by energy healers. The psychic shield I channeled from The Source back in 2011 still proves to be robust, repeatable, and efficient and can be downloaded from the correspondence course pages of my website (www.beyondthesource.org).

The location of the major chakras, English and Hindu names, their associated physical organs, their energetic templates, and their appearance are illustrated below. Please note that the colors used are NOT indicative of the true representation of the chakras or energetic templates because the colors used are for demarcation purposes only and are associated with the visible frequential spectrum of the human eye. True color representations of their energies are not possible for the incarnate human to perceive and as a result everything appears iridescent and colorless but with a tangible energy signature associated with them to allow the healer to discern the correct frequency level. Further below are some illustrations of chakra locations, damaged chakras, and forms of protection used on both the first and second level.

## Chakra Descriptions, Locations, and Anatomical Associations

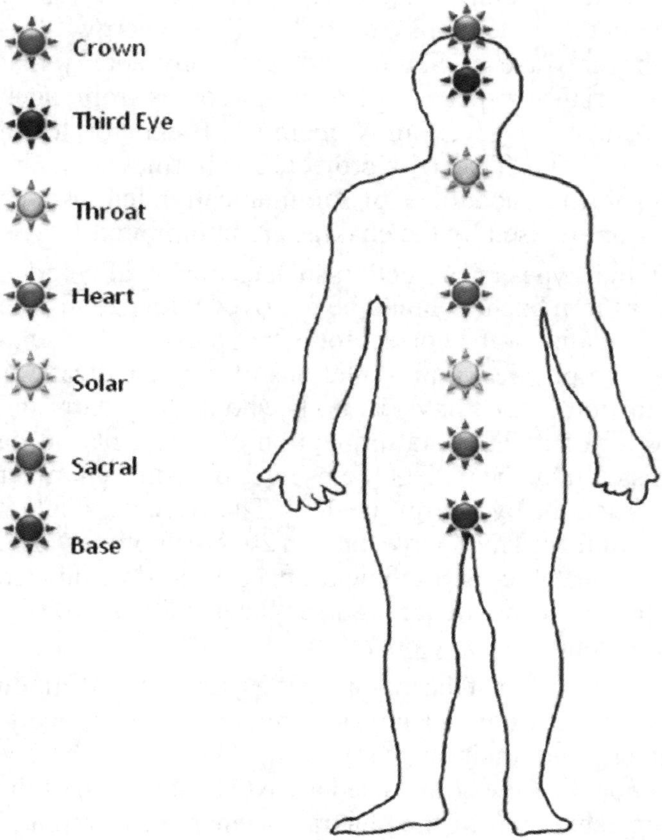

| | Level Number | English | Indian | Illustrative Color | | Anatomical Association | |
|---|---|---|---|---|---|---|---|
| | First | Base or Root | Muladhara | Red | Groin Area | Adrenals: Spinal Column, Kidneys | Vertically-Pointing toward the floor away from you |
| | Second | Sacral | Svadhishthana | Orange | 3" (7.5 cm) below the naval area | Gonads: Reproductive System | Horizontally - Pointing away from you |
| | Third | Solar | Manipura | Yellow | 3" (7.5 cm) above the naval area | Pancreas: Stomach, Liver, Gall Bladder, Nervous System | Horizontally - Pointing away from you |
| | Fourth | Heart | Anahata | Green | Sternum - 3" (7.5 cm) above the area where the left-and right- hand side of the chest join together | Thymus: Heart, Blood, Vagus Nerve, Circulatory System | Horizontally - Pointing away from you |
| | Fifth | Throat | Vishuddha | Blue | Middle of the throat | Thyroid: Bronchial & Vocal System, Lungs, Alimentary Canal | Horizontally - Pointing away from you |
| | Sixth | Third Eye | Ajna | Indigo | 3rd or spiritual eye, above bridge of the nose, inbetween the eyebrows | Pituitary: Lower Brain, Left Eye, Ears, Nose, Nervous System | Horizontally - Pointing away from you |
| | Seventh | Crown or Head | Sahasrara | Violet | Top of the crown of the head | Pineal: Upper Brain, Right Eye | Vertically-Pointing upward away from you |

Adapted from Barbara Brennan, *Hands of Light* (Bantam Books, 1987), Fig 7-5, p. 48; Guy Needler, *Traversing the Frequencies Workshops*, 2012-2020.

## Energy Template Descriptions and Functions

| | Level No. | Energy Templates | | |
|---|---|---|---|---|
| | | Layer Name | Appearance | Function |
| | 1st | Etheric Body | A web of tiny blue energy lines | An energy matrix or template of the physical body |
| | 2nd | Emotional Layer | Colored clouds in continual fluid motion | Displays and allows communication of the emotional content or feelings of love, joy, anger, etc. |
| | 3rd | Mental Body | Sturctured bright yellow light emanating from the head and shoulders of the body | Contains the structure of our thoughts and ideas |
| | 4th | Astral Level | Amorphous clouds of color infused with rose-colored light | Facilitates the transition of spiritual energy to physical energy and physcal energy to spiritual energy. Love between two people is displayed within this level |
| | 5th | Etheric Template | Has the appearance of a blue photograph negative made of cobalt blue lines | The blue print of perfect form for the etheric body to fill |
| | 6th | Celestial Body | Shimmering light made up of pastel colors with a gold silver shine | The communication of unconditional love and of "being one with God" |
| | 7th | Ketheric Template | A highly structured matrix of tiny gold-silver threads of light within an egg shape that shows the structure of the physical body and all chakras | Accumulation of past life bands, life plan, holds the Auric bodies together |
| | 8th-10th | No Names Identified | Gossamer-like structure increasing in fineness the higher one goes and finalizing in no structure | Main communication/link to the true and fully energetic self |

Adapted from Barbara Brennan, *Hands of Light* (Bantam Books, 1987), ch. 7, 41-56; Guy Needler, *Traversing the Frequencies Workshops*, 2012-2020.

# Organ or Body Part Reconstruction

Apart from conducting a basic chelation, organ and/ or body part reconstruction is one of the most common healing functions I perform. Whether it is aligned to a psycho-spiritual aspect of dysfunction or simply a physical manifestation, or not, I perform an organ and/ or body part reconstruction of some level in almost 95 percent of my healing work.

Organ and body part reconstruction needs to be performed on all seven levels associated with the gross physical and spirituo-physical aspects of the incarnate human vehicle. It cannot and should not be performed on just one level in isolation or more than one level but lower than seven frequency levels therefore leaving one or more frequency levels out.

In the event that the healer only works on reconstructing one or more of the lower frequency aspects of an organ or body part, its physical manifestations may initially disappear but they will ultimately return as the lower energetic templates are reprogrammed by the higher frequency templates. As the process behind both organ and body part (or even whole body) reconstruction is the same, for simplicity's sake I will focus on an organ.

## Perceiving the Organ to Be Reconstructed

It is important to first understand whether or not the organ is being affected from an external issue, such as a foreign object, or dysfunction due to energetic disharmony from the overall energetic template structure that creates the incarnate human vehicle before focusing in on the need to reconstruct the organ in question as the subject of the healing. This can be established by the healer elevating their frequencies to each of the seven levels individually and with their clairvoyance observing the whole picture of the energetic templates at each level, observing any overall issues that are directed toward the organ in question. The organ will appear to be represented in a solid fashion similar to that which is seen in the gross physical with the human eyes on each of the frequencies but will lack vibrancy and normal iridescent appearance (the main indicator of dysfunction). Overall issues should be dealt with from a total body template perspective. Foreign objects should be removed as a separate operation within the overall healing or as a specialized and focused healing in its own right. Foreign objects will be fully discussed in their own chapter.

Psycho-spiritual issues should also be taken into account and can be established during the initial appointment and the consultation performed with the patient.

Once the healer has established that the organ's function is not the result of external factors, the healer can focus on the need to either repair the energetic templates of the organ being healed or decide that they are to be totally replaced. Based upon this, organ reconstruction has two areas of healing to be considered. One, the repair of the energetic template/s associated with the organ. This may only require the need for one or more organ template levels to be repaired. Two, the total replacement of the energetic templates associated with the organ on all seven levels.

The repair of a specific organ template, although it may be seen as an isolated area of healing, needs to be considered in the light of the organ as a whole and as such the healer needs to check each template of the organ on each of the seven frequencies before embarking on repairing just one or two templates. If there is damage found on four or fewer templates, the healer will only need to repair those templates. If there appears to be five or more templates that need repairing, then the healer should move toward the need to replace all seven templates in totality.

Repairing an organ template can be achieved in the same way as repairing any part of the overall energetic templates associated with the incarnate human vehicle previously described. It is just that the healer is focusing on a function of the overall energetic template of the incarnate human vehicle and not a specific template in totality.

It is not necessary to replace a single template associated with an organ. Usually they can be repaired if fewer than four are damaged in some way. Reconstruction of an organ is therefore classified as such when all of the templates of the organ are in need of work and therefore need to be replaced.

## Replacing the Templates of the Organ

Having established that the organ needs all seven templates to be replaced, the healer should prepare to move between each of the seven frequencies quickly to allow the removal and replacement of the energetic templates. I should note here that one needs to think in terms of removing each template one by one and then when all templates are removed, cleansing the area of the organ and replacing them one by one. Removing and replacing a template and then moving onto the next can result in the new template being contaminated energetically by the old templates even if they are about to be replaced. This is because the integration between the templates is instantaneous and dysfunction can therefore be reestablished at the point of insertion of the new template.

Note that when replacing all of the templates associated with a specific organ, the healer should use their intention to hold the functionality of the overall set of energetic templates within an energy of functional stasis until the work on replacing the templates associated with the organ is completed. In this way, the healer maintains the energetic health of the patient throughout the duration of the organ reconstruction.

To remove the templates the healer needs to start at the first frequency level, which is associated with the root chakra, working their way up the frequencies. Once on this level, the healer can visualize the organ being connected to the overall energetic template of the incarnate human vehicle at this level by one or more connectors. I personally visualize two electrical connectors, one at each end of the organ. Each connector has an opposing connector specific to the organ in the same location within the overall energetic template. This allows the connectivity of the organ to the overall template at a specific frequency to be established, making the energetic template of the organ function correctly within the total functionality of the overall energetic template. Disconnect each of the connectors of the organ and remove the energetic template of the organ from the overall energetic template. Visualize your recycling bin. Place the old template within it to have its energy recycled by The Source. Cleanse the area with silver light, the properties of which having been previously described. Move onto the next level, the second level, and perform the same task. Move onto the remaining levels and do the same. Once all seven organ templates have been removed and their energies recycled by The Source, the healer can then move down to the first frequency level, which is associated with the root chakra, and start the replacement of the templates.

Visualize a new template, together with new connectors.

Place the new template of the organ in the location the old template was removed from and connect each of the connectors to the organ. Observe the template. Once the template is connected, you will see it start to glow iridescently. This indicates that it is functioning correctly.

Move onto the next level, the third level. Visualize a new template together with new connectors and perform the same task. Again, correct function will be illustrated by its appearance in an iridescent way. Move on to the remaining levels and do the same. Once all seven organ templates have been replaced, you will see that the overall image of the organ illustrates iridescence and vibrant energy. Also notice the appearance of the overall energetic templates of the incarnate human body at all seven frequency levels. Its appearance will also illustrate iridescence and vibrancy.

The healer can now remove their intention from maintaining the energetic stasis of the patient.

Provided that the patient is dedicated to working with the healer and is not intent on creating the same conditions that caused the organ to operate in a dysfunctional way in the first instance, the organ, or indeed any other part of the incarnate human vehicle that has been reconstructed, will return to is normal operating functionality. In essence, it will be healed.

# Past Life Trauma Healing (and Link Removal)

Past life trauma is a problem, psycho-spiritual or energetic, that we bring in from a previous or a number of previous incarnations or lives into this current life or incarnation. It is not limited to traumatic issues associated with past or parallel incarnations into the human vehicle and as a result can have the complications of coming with us from incarnations into other incarnate vehicles that we have used in previous incarnations on/into other planets, galaxies, and frequencies that we have had within the physical universe.

The fact that we can bring into this incarnation issues or energies that have traumatized us from other planets, galaxies, and frequencies can be easily missed. This results in the possibility that the healer fails to heal the patient correctly or provide a long-term healing solution.

How can a healer miss a past life trauma that has come from an incarnation in a different incarnate vehicle, on a different planet, in a different frequency?

Well, it's all about the depth of questioning that is applied by the healer during the initial or other consultation stage/s that the healer has with the patient. In general, a healer will be focusing on the human aspect of the patient in quite a linear way. First, the healer will look at the physical aspects of the patient that need healing. This will be purely from the perspective of the gross physical aspect of the incarnate human vehicle. Second, the healer will look at the energetics behind it, maybe looking into the energetic templates, organs/limbs, and possibly the human energy field or the human aura. Third, if the healer is experienced, they will look into the possibilities of past life issues with other incarnate individuals or their own experiences that they have had on the Earth. Fourth, they may look at the links that have been created between the Aspects or Shards that were part of the creation of the past life "incarnation" and the patient. It is possible that the healer will not consider the karmic aspects of the links or consider the possible fact that the past life trauma is not based upon the patient's incarnations on Earth but in other incarnate vehicle/s on other planet/s in other galaxy/ies in other frequency/ies within the physical universe.

Based upon this, the patient needs to be both questioned and scanned by the healer using the following questions to ensure that past life traumas are properly diagnosed, administered, dealt with, or healed.

- What needs to be healed?
    a. Is it physical?
    b. Is it psychological?
- What are the patient's thoughts on what is physically ailing them?
    a. Organs?
    b. Limbs?
    c. Nervous system?
    d. Endocrine system?
    e. Skeletal structure?
- What are the patient's thoughts on what is affecting them from a psychological perspective? How do they feel?
    a. Do they have family issues?
        i. Parents?
        ii. Siblings?
        iii. "In-Laws"?
        iv. Previous marriage partners?

v. Previous marriage children?
vi. Previous marriage "in-laws"?

b. Do they have issues with their partner?
c. Do they have issues with their children?
d. Do they have issues with work colleagues?
e. Do they have issues with friends?
f. Are they depressed?
g. Are they experiencing anxiety?
h. Are they experiencing tiredness?
i. Are they experiencing extremes in emotional responses?
j. Are they experiencing problems with temper or calmness?
k. Are they experiencing problems with ownership/responsibility?

Once the healer has worked with these questions and recognized that the issue/s the patient is facing is/are not attributed to this incarnation, only then can they consider a past life association or trauma.

Having understood that the patient needs to be healed based upon a past life trauma the healer needs to meditate on the patient, allowing them to answer the following additional questions:

1. Is there a link with a previous method of demise?
   a. Can the healer see (with their mind's or spiritual [third] eye) energies associated with the demise of the previous incarnate vehicle?
      i. Was the demise associated with accident?
         1. Was the demise associated with fire?
         2. Was the demise associated with water?
         3. Was the demise associated with

disease?
4. Was the demise associated with being crushed?

b. Do the energies represent demise via aggression?
   i. Torture?
   ii. Weapon?
   iii. Execution?
2. Is the link with another individual?
3. Is this link Earth based?
4. Is the link based within another environment?
   a. Planet?
   b. Galaxy?
   c. Frequency?

Once the healer has asked all of these questions and received intuition about which of these questions, or which combination of these questions, and answers apply, only then can the healer focus in on the origin of the past life trauma and effect a robust healing that is going to last and not require the patient to return for more healing.

The healer now has a focal point. This being:

- The issue is based upon a past life trauma.
- The past life trauma is based upon a method of demise.
- The past life trauma is based upon the relationship with another incarnate entity.
- The physical location of the past life trauma is known.
- The frequential level of the past life trauma is known.
- Whether or not there is karma involved.

The healer is now fully equipped to heal the patient! Armed with all of the answers to the questions above, the healer now has to connect with the patient by raising their own frequencies to that of the seventh level by opening all of their chakras one by one. This will allow the healer to connect with the past life trauma issues on all seven levels concurrently, negating the need to work on one level and then the next level, and so on.

## Removing the Past Life Trauma

In the event that the past life trauma is based upon an aggressive method of demise, the healer will now be able to actively "see" with their mind's eye the method of aggression. As with previous methods of demise being a function of demise by weapon, the healer can now place themselves on the seventh frequency level and ask to be shown the circumstances that led to the demise by weapon and what weapon was used. The healer can also ask whether that weapon was based upon the Earth or another planet/frequency or if any karmic links have been made with the incarnate individual who used the weapon.

In the event that is simply a matter of demise by aggressive use of weapon and that the incarnate Aspect of the patient was actively participating in some event or other that resulted in the use of a weapon, the healer can use the method explained in the chapter about removing foreign objects from a chakra to remove the energies of the weapon from the energies of the energetic templates, which may include a chakra, of the patient.

Once the energy/ies of the weapon is/are removed, the healer then needs to remove the link between the patient and the incarnation of the Aspect of the patient in the past life in question to ensure that the trauma does not reoccur and cause the patient physical dysfunction and psycho-spiritual issues based around the same theme.

## Removing Past Life Links

Having established that there is a link to a past life

and that the link to the method of demise, experience, or psychological issue is based upon or within this life, irrespective of whether it is on the Earth or another location/frequency then the healer can work to sever that link.

I do have to note here that some healers who know how to sever a link generally only do that and miss the fact that this link can, and normally does, reestablish itself upon a later date. Based upon this, the healer needs to not only remove the link, but also the method of linking both at the location of the current incarnation and the location, environment, and frequency of the previous incarnation. The healer can perform this task from the seventh frequency level by opening the chakras as previously mentioned.

While on the seventh level, the healer needs to visualize the patient within an incarnate vehicle in both the current incarnation and the incarnation creating the issue. The healer will see a link, an energy line, between some part of the incarnate human vehicle in this incarnation and the incarnate vehicle that is the focus of the past life trauma.

The healer should also visualize the recycling bin used in previous descriptions.

Although I visualize the link between the two incarnations as being an electric cable with a plug on either end of the cable, it is clearly an energetic link. This link connects the individual's Event Space with the past life/incarnation and the current Event Space and life/incarnation. The link is connected to the energies of the incarnate vehicles used in both Event Spaces by the stress, trauma, or profundity of the incarnation at the point of, or close to, the demise of the previous incarnate vehicle and the current incarnate vehicle by the focus of the Aspect on the experience during the intensity of the moment of the experience. It manifests as a lump of energy on each of the seven energetic/frequential templates integrating them in an adaptive way with the link and the seven energetic/frequential templates of the past and current incarnation.

## Illustrations of the Locations of Links with Other Incarnations

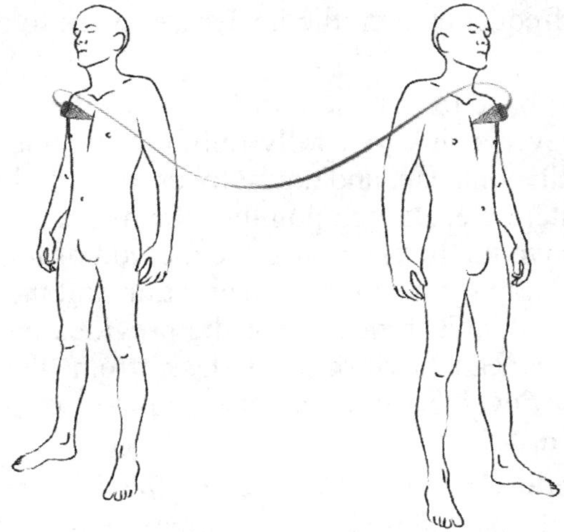

Links between the Heart Chakra

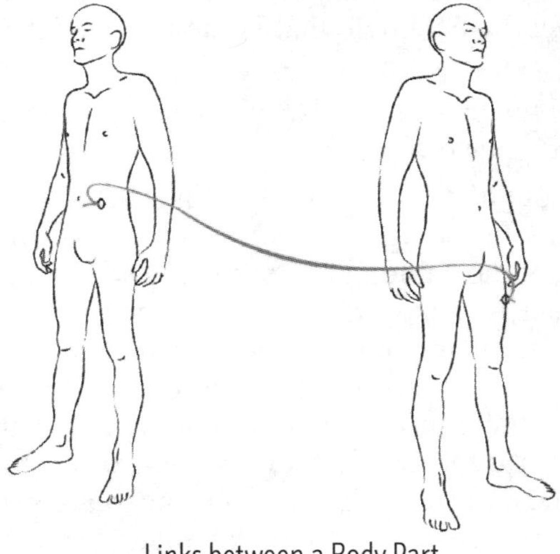

Links between a Body Part

Using my illustration, each plug is connected to a socket on the body of each incarnate vehicle, rather like an electric socket on the wall of your house.

Visualize removing the plug (connection) from each end of the cable (link) from the socket on the body of the incarnate vehicle of the patient in this current incarnation and the incarnation that has been identified as the one that is affecting the current incarnation. Deposit the cable and plugs into your energy recycling bin. This simply severs the link between the past life (incarnation) and the current incarnation. However, as stated above it only severs the link and not the connectivity. If the connectivity between the incarnations is not removed as well, the link can be reestablished, recreating the issues that were previously invoked by such a link.

Continuing to use the theme of the electrical plugs, cable, and wall socket to remove the link, the healer should now concentrate on removing the sockets on the bodies of the current and past life. I use the visualization of unscrewing the faceplate of the socket and then removing the wires from the faceplate before terminating the wires correctly in an electrically secure way such as using terminal blocks (a way of connecting electrical wires together) and wrapping insulation tape around them. I then visualize backfilling the remaining hole with energy so that the hole no longer exists. If one uses the visualization of filling the patras (where the socket is embedded into the wall) with plaster, as in the example that the socket was on a wall in your house, then you have created a solid block of energy that stops the possibility of reconnecting with the past life. Provided, that is, that both sockets on the patient and their past life are solidly backfilled, there is no way that a new connection or link can be created.

Clearly this is only one method of visualizing the link between the incarnations. Other methods can be created and personalized according to the working practices and imagination of the healer to achieve the same thing.

Common links to past lives that have an effect on the current incarnation of the patient can be based upon the following themes:

- **Accident**: such as house fire, drowning, electrocution from household device or wiring, falling from a horse, falling over and banging the head on a rock with the incarnate suffering brain damage or a broken neck. There are myriad accidents that can be traumatic with that trauma being passed on to the next incarnation or other downstream incarnations. Transportation-based accidents such as demise by car, train, boat, or plane crash can create a common theme for a past life link. The method of how we demise can profoundly affect us in one of our next lives.
- **Aggressive interaction**: such as the incarnation being terminated as a result of war or being attacked by a stranger or adversary either individually or with a group of people, execution, rape, torture.
- **Environment**: can be defined as natural disaster. Demise via earthquake, tsumani, wind/storm (hurricane, tornado, cyclone), volcano, bush fire, flood.
- **Disease**: has a number of genetic and transmitted functions such as cancers, heart or lung disease (cystic fibrosis), AIDS, cholera, measles, mumps, leprosy, chicken and small pox, yellow fever, malaria, and influenza to name a few.
- **Circumstance**: includes being a bystander, hostage, loss of employment, loss of partner, social environment, homelessness, poverty, education, and crime.
- **Addiction**: to drugs, alcohol, tobacco, foods, low frequency thoughts, behaviors, and actions, control and coercion, aggressive thoughts and actions, material wealth and status, masochism, sadism. These are all creations of the feeling of power, release, or

distraction from why we incarnate.

- **Universal/frequential location**: a desire to incarnate into certain locations on the Earth where certain thought and behavior patterns are acceptable or a desire to be in a certain environment every time the Aspect incarnates.
- **Psychological/psycho-spiritual**: depression, stress, anxiety, poor me, subversion, betrayal, sexual abuse can and do supress our ability to function in a clear and coherent way.
- **Karmic link**: a link to a need to repay a karmic debt with another Aspect, the so-called need to receive or administer that which was received or administered by/to the Aspect the karmic link is with. The need to remove a desire to experience sensory stimulus/pleasures or the need to change the way one interacts or reacts with a certain experience or interaction with others. This creates an efficient incarnation and meaningful interaction with one's peers and the environment.
- **Parallel lives**: affect us at times when we have visions of alternative locations and experiences that we cannot relate to normally. When we have a link to a parallel life, we struggle to relate to what is supposed to be the focus of our attention in this incarnation because there appears to be a conflict in the continuity of our chain of experience. The logical start or end of an experience or series of experiences are not present and so creates confusion. A link with a parallel life or existence can be misdiagnosed as psychosis, schizophrenia, or other psychological issues. Severing the link with a parallel life or existence restores the focus on this incarnation reducing/removing confusion and creating a more grounded individual.

With the plethora of ways in which our previous incarnations can affect us in this incarnation, should we let them, it is not surprising that many physical and psychological issues that we face are created as a function of remembering on an energetic level that which brought us pain in a past life or the demise of that life.

# Psychic Surgery

Psychic surgery is the use of energies or entities to assist in, perform, or complete the healing of a patient with the view to healing an issue that is creating what appears to be a physical disease, or dysfunction in the gross physical Aspect of the physical universe focused upon the Earth; in essence, to perform the energetic version of a physical medical response.

Psychic surgery has, in my mind, three main ways of being actioned.

The first way is the use of the hands to physically enter the body of the patient using specific techniques to remove the matter that is creating the illness. This is normally attributed to the removal of tumors or dysfunctional aspects of an organ. There is usually the presentation of some blood in this method along with the fleshy component of the tumor or dysfunctional organ. As I have no experience of this method of psychic surgery, I will not be describing how to perform it. Neither do I advocate anyone practicing it without in-depth instruction and continued coaching.

The second way is based upon energy healing and so falls within the content taught to me by my healing instructor and the experiences I have had in using this particular healing modality.

In energy healing, one does not perform psychic surgery per se; one invokes the area for psychic surgery to be performed by another entity. In essence, the energy healer can either accept the help of another entity, should it be offered, or they can request the help of an entity.

The entities that I, and my energy healing colleagues, have encountered tend to be specialized to one or a number of related healing subjects and it is quite possible that the healer may never experience the benefit of a certain healing entity more than once in their career.

## An Offer of Help

An offer of help may be presented to the healer if they are about to face a difficult healing such as one that they do not have a healing modality to apply. In this instance, while the healer is visualizing the work necessary to affect a healing, an entity may present itself to the healer offering their services, which may be presented to the healer as a specialized healing function that the healer is not aware of or capable of administering. Alternatively, if an entity does not make themselves available, then the healer can make a request for help as specified below.

## A Request for Help

A request for help ultimately results in the offer of help from a number of entities that have the specialist skills requested by the healer.

To make a request for help, the healer simply needs to use their desire to receive help in the healing work that they are doing to attract the attention of a healing entity.

If the healer has a desire to attract the attention of a healing entity, then the most basic method is to use a short mantra to assist them in the broadcasting.

A suggested example is illustrated below:

1. I desire the help of a specialized healing entity.
    - One that is specialized in XXXX
2. I desire the help of a specialized healing entity.
    - One that is specialized in XXXX
3. I desire the help of a specialized healing entity.

- One that is specialized in XXXX

And so on. Repeat these twelve times.

XXXX can be brain surgery, replacing the endocrine system, osteopathy, or any other medical specialism.

The number twelve is significant because it is associated with the dominant aspect of the structure of The Origin, The Source Entity, and therefore us as smaller individualized units of The Source. Because of this, repeating one's desire twelve times makes a significant impression upon the desire of the healer and his/her broadcast for help in healing a needy patient.

Note that in broadcasting the healer's desire for help, they may be exposing themselves to the possibility that a high intelligence astral entity will take the opportunity to approach them. As a result, they will need to be discerning and use their intuition to judge whether or not the entity is a direct creation of Source, that being, an Aspect of a True Energetic Self (TES). If not, it may be an astral entity posing as a healing entity to gain energy from the healer or the patient. The healer should use their power as a direct individualization of their TES, which is a direct individualization of The Source to use a psychic shield to protect themselves and the patient so that astral entities cannot take advantage of the open desire of the healer to accept help. Once the healer has ascertained that the entity is pure of action, thought, and intention, healing intention, then they can allow the entity to work on their patient. The entity may not use healing modalities or techniques that are known to incarnate mankind (yet) and so may appear to be something else other than healing. It is generally best to allow the entity to carry on with their work until the healer is invited to take over. It is quite common to be asked to hold the energy. This means that the healer is required to work on holding the frequency around the patient and the space that they are working within, usually a room in the house they live in or a room within a healing establishment, at a high level until the work is completed. The healer can achieve a higher level of frequency by using the chakra opening exercises previously described. However, they need to be used with the minor exception that the healer also needs to use their intention (or mentally spoken word) to allow the energies associated with them when opening the chakras to permeate throughout the venue used to perform their healings as well as the patient themselves. The healer therefore needs to increase the frequencies or "hold the energy" for the psychic surgeon, the healing entity, and the location to be able to come to a frequency that is high enough for it to work on the patient. In effect, the healing entity, the psychic surgeon, can only come down to a certain frequency level, no lower than the middle of the fourth frequency, before it is unable to operate in an efficient way. It is because of this that the healer, in raising the frequencies by their intention to be of service, raises the frequency of the healing space and the patient to the level where the entity that is to help can help.

Also, the point of raising the frequencies of the patient and the healing space is to allow those entities that have gained some skills in the healing arts to get as close to the patient as possible so as to allow them to check the work that they have performed on the patient in the gross physical. If you remember that disincarnate entities exist in the energetic structure of The Source, then you will realize that the healing entity, who may well be providing a healing art function that is above the fourth frequency, will need to understand what the healer intended to heal and will need to check the work that it had done on behalf of the healer.

## Copying the Work of a Physical Surgeon

In the third way, the healer mirrors the work of a physical surgeon while visualizing the repair of an organ or limb, or even the transplantation of an organ or limb. They may even visualize an operating theater and the support of nurses. In this method, it is not uncommon for an Aspect that was incarnate as a doctor or consultant or consultant surgeon to offer assistance or request/suggest that they take over the management of and administration of the surgery necessary to heal the patient.

# Auric Layer Reconstruction

The human energy field or human aura provides an essential function of protection from energetic attacks, coercion, and astral entities. It also protects the incarnate human aspect from low frequency energies that can adhere to us like dust or an amoeba or like jelly covering a mould.

Low frequency energies that manifest as dust or an amoeba or jelly are discussed in astral entity removal because they are essentially the start of the evolution of energy to the point where they begin to create rudimentary intelligence and become an astral entity.

When the aura is damaged, the protection from the low frequency energies is impaired and the low frequency energies can infiltrate this natural protection by clogging up the chakras and sticking to the energetic templates creating energetic imbalance and physical dysfunction.

Reconstruction of the auric layers has to be performed one layer at a time and on the frequency level associated with that auric level.

The auric layers have many images associated with them in spiritual texts, quite a number of of which even give them colors. However, they are essentially colorless due to the fact that they are frequentially higher than those frequencies sensed by the physical human eye, which we perceive as color, and as a result we suggest that the layers of the human energy field have colors attributed to them, when in fact they do not. The auric layers being colorless are best perceived by their structure, which changes as a function of the frequencies they are associated with.

The structure of each of the auric layers changes according to their frequency; however, they can be visualized as the same basic structure for ease of repair. This basic structure can be seen to be similar to a fishing net, of the type used by trawlers, wrapped around the body in the shape of an egg or rugby football. Each of the layers will be, in general, spaced about 25 mm away from each other. Although this is a general rule of thumb the auric layers of a patient that lives in a busy city will be closer together than those auric layers of a patient who lives in the countryside.

To repair the auric layers, the healer must use the chakra opening exercise described at the start of this book, extending and rotating clockwise each chakra one by one until all seven layers have been repaired.

Before commencing the work of repairing the auric layers, the healer should scan each of the layers in turn. This ensures that the healer can see which layers need repairing and which do not.

To help the healer to repair the auric layers in a repeatable and robust way, I suggest the following process:

- Ground both yourself and the patient by using your intention to be grounded. (This will assist in the recovery process of the patient after the work has been done because they will not be so tired.)
- Visualize an energetic link between you as the healer and the patient. This will ensure that your intention to move through the frequencies to work on the auric layers will also include your patient.
- Open the root or base chakra by extending it to its largest size and rotate it clockwise. This brings you up to the first frequency layer.
- Using your visualization (clairvoyance) via

your third or spiritual eye, scan the entire auric layer from top to bottom, left to right, and front to back in a circular motion. Record the location/s of any tears or rips in the net-like structure of the layer at this first level. (Remember that the third or spiritual eye is not the third or spiritual eye chakra. Although they are in the same location on the forehead, they are entirely different things.)

- Open the sacral chakra by extending it to its largest size and rotate it clockwise. This brings you up to the second frequency layer.
- Using your visualization (clairvoyance) via your third or spiritual eye, scan the entire auric layer from top to bottom, left to right, and front to back in a circular motion. Record the location/s of any tears or rips in the net-like structure of the layer at this second level.
- Open the solar chakra by extending it to its largest size and rotate it clockwise. This brings you up to the third frequency layer.
- Using your visualization (clairvoyance) via your third or spiritual eye, scan the entire auric layer from top to bottom, left to right, and front to back in a circular motion. Record the location/s of any tears or rips in the net-like structure of the layer at this third level.
- Open the heart chakra by extending it to its largest size and rotate it clockwise. This brings you up to the fourth frequency layer.
- Using your visualization (clairvoyance) via your third or spiritual eye, scan the entire auric layer from top to bottom, left to right, and front to back in a circular motion. Record the location/s of any tears or rips in the net-like structure of the layer at this fourth level.

- Open the throat chakra by extending it to its largest size and rotate it clockwise. This brings you up to the fifth frequency layer.
- Using your visualization (clairvoyance) via your third or spiritual eye, scan the entire auric layer from top to bottom, left to right, and front to back in a circular motion. Record the location/s of any tears or rips in the net-like structure of the layer at this fifth level.
- Open the third or spiritual eye chakra by extending it to its largest size and rotate it clockwise. This brings you up to the sixth frequency layer.
- Using your visualization (clairvoyance) via your third or spiritual eye, scan the entire auric layer from top to bottom, left to right, and front to back in a circular motion. Record the location/s of any tears or rips in the net-like structure of the layer at this sixth level.
- Open the crown chakra by extending it to its largest size and rotate it clockwise. This brings you up to the seventh frequency layer.
- Using your visualization (clairvoyance) via your third or spiritual eye, scan the entire auric layer from top to bottom, left to right, and front to back in a circular motion. Record the location/s of any tears or rips in the net-like structure of the layer at this seventh level.

Close all of the chakras. This can be achieved in the following ways:

- Stop the rotation of the crown chakra and contract it into its point of origin. This brings you down to the sixth frequency level.
- Stop the rotation of the third or spiritual eye

chakra and contract it into its point of origin. This brings you down to the fifth frequency level.

- Stop the rotation of the throat chakra and contract it into its point of origin. This brings you down to the fourth frequency level.
- Stop the rotation of the heart chakra and contract it into its point of origin. This brings you down to the third frequency level.
- Stop the rotation of the solar chakra and contract it into its point of origin. This brings you down to the second frequency level.
- Stop the rotation of the sacral chakra and contract it into its point of origin. This brings you down to the first frequency level.
- Stop the rotation of the base or root chakra and contract it into its point of origin. This brings you down to the Earth or base frequency level.

Follow this process to repair the auric layers at each level:

- Open the root or base chakra by extending it to its largest size and rotate it clockwise. This brings you up to the first frequency layer.
- Using your visualization (clairvoyance) via your third or spiritual eye, visualize repairing the tears or rips in the net-based structure by inserting energy lines between the lines that are disconnected. See how the auric layer at this first layer changes its appearance and becomes iridescent when all tears/rips are repaired.
- Open the sacral chakra by extending it to its largest size and rotate it clockwise. This brings you up to the second frequency layer.

- Using your visualization (clairvoyance) via your third or spiritual eye, visualize repairing the tears or rips in the net-based structure by inserting energy lines between the lines that are disconnected. See how the auric layer at this second layer changes its appearance and becomes iridescent when all tears/rips are repaired.
- Open the solar chakra by extending it to its largest size and rotate it clockwise. This brings you up to the third layer.
- Using your visualization (clairvoyance) via your third or spiritual eye, visualize repairing the tears or rips in the net-based structure by inserting energy lines between the lines that are disconnected. See how the auric layer at this third layer changes its appearance and becomes iridescent when all tears/rips are repaired.
- Open the heart chakra by extending it to its largest size and rotate it clockwise. This brings you up to the fourth frequency layer.
- Using your visualization (clairvoyance) via your third or spiritual eye, visualize repairing the tears or rips in the net-based structure by inserting energy lines between the lines that are disconnected. See how the auric layer at this fourth layer changes its appearance and becomes iridescent when all tears/rips are repaired.
- Open the throat chakra by extending it to its largest size and rotate it clockwise. This brings you up to the fifth frequency layer.
- Using your visualization (clairvoyance) via your third or spiritual eye, visualize repairing the tears or rips in the net-based structure by

inserting energy lines between the lines that are disconnected. See how the auric layer at this fifth layer changes its appearance and becomes iridescent when all tears/rips are repaired.

- Open the third or spiritual eye chakra by extending it to its largest size and rotate it clockwise. This brings you up to the sixth frequency layer.
- Using your visualization (clairvoyance) via your third or spiritual eye, visualize repairing the tears or rips in the net-based structure by inserting energy lines between the lines that are disconnected. See how the auric layer at this sixth layer changes its appearance and becomes iridescent when all tears/rips are repaired.
- Open the crown chakra by extending it to its largest size and rotate it clockwise. This brings you up to the seventh frequency layer.
- Using your visualization (clairvoyance) via your third or spiritual eye, visualize repairing the tears or rips in the net-based structure by inserting energy lines between the lines that are disconnected. See how the auric layer at this seventh layer changes its appearance and becomes iridescent when all tears/rips are repaired.

Close all of the chakras. This can be achieved in the following ways:

- Stop the rotation of the crown chakra and contract it into its point of origin. This brings you down to the sixth frequency level.
- Stop the rotation of the third or spiritual eye

chakra and contract it into its point of origin. This brings you down to the fifth frequency level.

- Stop the rotation of the throat chakra and contract it into its point of origin. This brings you down to the fourth frequency level.
- Stop the rotation of the heart chakra and contract it into its point of origin. This brings you down to the third frequency level.
- Stop the rotation of the solar chakra and contract it into its point of origin. This brings you down to the second frequency level.
- Stop the rotation of the sacral chakra and contract it into its point of origin. This brings you down to the first frequency level.
- Stop the rotation of the base or root chakra and contract it into its point of origin. This brings you down to the Earth or base frequency level.

The healer can now remove the grounding from the patient and themselves.

It is beneficial for the healer to step back and observe the patient from a distance with the patient standing in front of a white wall. By dis-focusing the physical eyes, the healer should now be able to see the difference in the appearance of the newly repaired auric field. It will appear fully iridescent and have the appearance of being in high definition as well. The healer will also be able to notice an overall change in the demeanor of the client, which will be more positive and friendly in nature.

# Astral Entity Removal

One of the most common forms of healing I administer to a patient is astral entity removal. Astral entities are a very common energetic parasite that, as previously described, can be created by the incarnate Aspect, usually subconsciously, or can develop as a function of Darwinian evolution of stray energy.

Almost every incarnate human on planet Earth has an astral entity attached to some part of themselves but are totally unaware of this fact or the feeling associated with having an astral entity attached to them.

This I feel is just as well. It's a blessing in disguise. If those of us that are in an immersed incarnation were to be exposed to the details of the greater reality at the levels outside of the visual range of the human eye, which includes the devices that have been developed to detect that which is just outside of the visual range, such as infrared and radio/microwave technology, then they would be horrified at best at what they could see. If one is educated and subsequently exposed to these realities in a gradual way, then there is no real problem. However, to suddenly know that one is being used by another entity for the energetic gain of that entity, and that it may use the hosts darkest fears to shield or hide itself, may well cause psychological problems.

As a result, and in the interests of the psychological health of the client or patient, the healer may need to test the knowledge of the client or patient before divulging the details of what they have found attached to them, and where they are attached in the post healing summary they may perform for the client or patient.

Astral entities are, to my mind, a plague. Astral entities can be found attached to one or more of the auric layers, having first ripped or torn all the auric layers before settling in on a layer or layers that they are comfortable with. They can also be found attached to one or more of the energetic templates, which also included those templates associated with the major physical organs. And, as previously discussed in the chapters on chakra healing, they can be found attached to one or more of your chakras.

To reiterate what astral entities are though:

Astral entities exist in the frequencies associated with the fourth, fifth, sixth, and seventh frequencies of our universal environment. The fourth is the lower astral; the fifth, the upper lower astral; the sixth, the lower upper astral; and the seventh, the upper astral. They mostly exist in the fourth and fifth frequencies though. They can only ascend to the sixth and seventh frequencies via the symbiotic work with a long-term host. However, they can go no further because they are in individual evolutionary stasis once they rely on the host for energy and its desire for its continued existence by the creating incarnate human, following the demise of the incarnate human vehicle, has no momentum.

Their existence, however, is mostly transitory because they cannot maintain their existence through the metabolization of their own energy. Therefore, they take energy from other, higher and usually incarnate, entities—hence being attached to the incarnate human vehicle and animal incarnate vehicles.

They are created in two ways, either by us as human beings as a function of desire, personal energetic attack, or adversarial thoughts aimed toward another, or by the normal evolution of energy coalescing together in a form of Darwinian evolution—mutual attraction to similar or same energy or frequency. Astral entities, however, only have a level of intelligence that revolves around their survival or perpetuated existence through the appropriation of energy from those entities or beings that are incarnate. Some of this intelligence is detailed enough to allow the astral entity to create a symbiotic relationship with an incarnate host by making them feel powerful or by controlling the host in some way. Others are simply low intelligence amoeba-like beings.

Note that I have used both the words "entity" and "being" to describe astral entities.

I will elaborate a little on what the difference is between an entity and a being for the sake of completeness.

- An "entity" is an individualized unit of sentience given a body of energy/ies by the division of sentience away from a higher entity, by that higher entity. Or, in the case of the astral entity is created by an entity using energies external to itself. However, they have no further ability to evolve due to the desire behind the intention to create them not being aligned to an evolutionary requirement. All in all, because they are not sentient they cannot be classified as an entity, even though they are created by a sentient entity.
- A "being" is an individualized unit of sentience that has developed independently by the function of similar, same, or sympathetic energy/ies collecting together and evolving over a period. Or, in the case of the astral entity, is not in the possession of sentience but is developing individual rudimentary intelligence through a similar or same route that would have eventually resulted in the creation of a sentient being. This being, had it not aligned itself to a host or is not dissolved by a healer or by The Source, may actually over a long period have developed sentience. Alignment to a host to gain energy places the individual development of a group of energies

into stasis as it stops the incentive to progress from an evolutionary perspective.

It can be seen therefore that we should call astral creations neither astral entities nor astral beings, the nomenclature use being a function of how they got to where they are functionality wise rather than sentience wise. However, for the sake of the common understanding I will continue to use the name astral entity to cover both means of creation.

There are many ways in which an astral entity attaches itself to a host other than via the chakras, the spinal column being a second favorite. All locations of attachment create mild to severe discomfort to the host.

In most cases, however, the person will become the host either as a result of the astral entity being the subject of the astral entity's creation, and use, as an attacking or adversarial medium, or through it being drawn to the potential host in its need to gain energy to perpetuate its existence as a result of the host having weak protection or having an overwhelming and strong and nondiscriminatory desire to communicate with a disincarnate spirit, which leaves them wide open to being a host.

When an astral entity is attached to any other part of the incarnate human vehicle other than a chakra, it can be manifest on any or all of the gross physical and spirituo-physical frequencies and as a result, the removal of that entity must be performed on a number of, or all seven, gross physical and spirituo-physical frequencies. However, it is normal for an astral entity to be predominantly associated with the frequencies of the energy template or auric layer that it is attached to, and not detected on the other frequency levels. If this is the case, then the astral entity only needs to be removed from the template or auric layer on that frequency that it is attached to and no other. I do have to say, though, that I have experienced a number of astral entities that are attached to the host on all seven levels. When this is the case, the astral entity is using the host's auric layers as a shield so that it is not perceived by the host or those who know and interact with the host.

Once the healer has established where the astral entity is taking energy from, the healer must open their own chakra/s to elevate themselves to the frequency of the frequency level/s that the entity is going to be removed from.

As previously stated, the astral entity normally tries to defend itself and may present a shape or form to the healer they find abhorrent or are fearful of. If this is the case, the healer must be aware that they are significantly more powerful than the astral entity and should not pay any attention to how big or fearful the image presented to the healer is. Any fear projected from the healer will be used against the healer by the astral entity and be projected back to them. The healer will then, in most cases, consider that the job of removing the entity is too big or difficult for them and will abandon the healing work. The astral entity therefore survives to exist for another day, so to speak.

A competent and well-trained healer will ignore any defensive responses by the astral entity and continue with the task of removal.

Once at the correct frequency, and observing the astral entity with their perception, the healer can then visualize removing the entity by taking full grip of the entity with both energetic hands.

Gently and firmly take hold of the entity in the same way as you might a wriggling cat from a friend or partner's lap, safely extracting the cat's claws from their clothing. As with the wriggling cat example, the astral entity may decide to "hang on" to the energetic templates of a physical organ so be prepared to move the entity around in a few angles of movement or employ a "third" energetic arm and hand or even enlist the help of a trusted entity that helps with healing such as a healing entity or your Guide or one of its Helpers to lend another hand. Again be careful not to cause damage to the energy template or auric layer by removing the astral entity. When you have teased the astral entity away from the energy template or auric layer, the healer can send the entity back to The Source Entity so that its energy can be recycled by The Source. This is achieved by visualizing the recycling bin as previously described and placing the entity within it.

In the event that the energy template or auric layer has sustained some damage as a result of removing the astral entity, the affected areas can be healed by using the techniques previously described.

I stated that in most cases an astral entity that is attached to a chakra is usually predominantly represented on the frequency of the energy template or auric layer that the entity is taking energy from. If this is not the case then the healer will need to establish, via scanning the patient, which of the remaining templates or auric layers are also affected and repeat this work on each of them one by one, including any potential repair work created by removing the entity.

It is also worth noting that if an astral entity is attached to more than one energy template of a physical organ, the healer is advised to work on removing the entity from the lowest frequency template, performing any repair work first, before moving on to the next highest frequency template. As the healer moves up the frequencies, they will notice that the work of removing the astral entity from the energy template or auric layer and performing any repair work becomes faster and faster the higher up the frequencies they progress.

Removal of an astral entity from a patient usually results in an immediate and positive response. If, however, this is not the case then the healer needs to revisit the "need to" scan the patient's energetic bodies to look for other, smaller entities that may have been missed and remove them as well.

## The Appearance of an Astral Entity Attached to an Energy Template

The best way to consider what an astral entity looks like when it is taking energy from one of your client's energetic templates is to experience it firsthand. The healer can do this by using their intention to use the function of their spiritual or third eye to scan the energy templates individually by opening their own chakras one by one and scanning the template associated with the chakra that is open, one by one. The astral entity will be perceived in the mind's eye in most instances. On some occasions, though, this may be experienced as an overlay on the vision seen through the physical eyes. Whichever way you as the healer see or perceive the energetic, the astral entity will appear or present itself in one of two main ways. The first way is, as previously explained, by the entity reading the mind of the host and presenting an image that the patient is frightened of, that they find abhorrent. The use of an abhorrent image is designed to make the host look the other way, so to speak, not wanting to see that which they find abhorrent as a method of distracting the host from looking closer at what they are seeing or perceiving. In this way, you the healer will also perceive the astral entity in the imagery that it has chosen to use as its main image of distraction with its host.

More often than not the astral entity is only perceivable on the frequencies that it predominantly exists within. However, it is also possible that the healer can perceive the astral entity on other frequency levels as well, specifically those that are next to, this means above and below, the frequency that the astral entity exists within. The healer will perceive an almost translucent or shadow image of the astral entity on the frequencies above and below the frequency that it exists within. It may even look blurred! In this instance, it will only be when the healer elevates his/her own frequencies to that which is the same as that of the astral entity that he/she will see the astral entity as a clearly defined and detailed image.

The second way is to see the astral entity as it really is, a mass of semi-intelligent energy that is interlocked or intertwined within the energies of the energetic templates. Again, it may be perceivable only on the energetic template that is associated with its own frequency of existence and may also be visible to some extent on those frequencies just above and below the dominant frequency of existence.

The third way is that the healer sees the astral entity as a function of their own fears and blockages. In this instance, the astral entity seeing and feeling a danger to its own existence reads the mind of the healer and presents back to the healer the images that they find abhorrent. An astral entity can even work with the ego of the healer, which is always looking for ways in which to keep the healer in frequencies lower than it is currently experiencing so that it can perpetuate its own existence. Remember this, the lower the frequency of the healer, the less effective that healer is! The astral entity, working in collaboration with the ego of the healer, can even make the healer think that he/she has removed the astral entity when in fact he/she has not. This is a very good example of why the healer needs to perform significant levels of psycho-spiritual work on him/herself under the strict guidance of an experienced healing teacher. This is a necessary requirement to ensure that the healer is, by and large, immune to such responses.

Each of the energetic templates can be considered as a three-dimensional (height, width, depth—not dimensional as in terms of the structure of the multiversal environment) matrix of frequency and energy that is used to create the basis for the incarnate human vehicle. The templates are overlaid upon each other within and occupying the same space but at frequencies that are independent of each other while being linked together by the lines of connectivity between the chakras. This self-same method is used to create other incarnate vehicles in other locations within the physical universe.

When an astral entity is attached to one of the seven energetic templates, it weaves itself into the template, making itself part of the template. In this way, an astral entity can maximize the amount of energy that it can take from the host by connecting itself to one of the energetic templates by increasing the area of integration or connectivity of its own energy body with the template in the process. This makes astral entities very difficult to be perceived and removed because the entity can even appear to "BE" the energy template as well; such is the potential level of integration available to the resourceful astral entity.

In the event that the astral entity attaches and integrates itself to two or more energetic templates, the work of the healer becomes even more difficult in terms of removal. Dealing with an astral entity that has integrated itself with two or more energy templates requires a healer of high level of experience and skill. One saving grace here, though, is that in the process of integrating with two or more energy templates, the astral entity actually makes itself more visible to the healer. This is because in integrating with two or more energy templates, the astral entity generates a link between the templates that it is integrated with, with its own energy body. This is easily seen by the healer as an energy breach between the frequencies associated with the energy templates affected. Additionally, not all of the astral entity is therefore located on one energy template so the level of integration on a particular template is not as complete, making the job of removing the astral entity easier on each of the energy templates than it would be if it was integrated within one energy template only.

I would like to make the point here that the energy template/s that the astral entity attaches itself to may be the whole energy template for a certain frequency level/levels or it can be just the energy template/s associated with a major physical organ or physical system such as the veins, blood, nervous system, skin, or skeleton. You as the healer therefore need to observe in a nonexpectant way (expectation creates an error and/or a blockage in how the healer perceives the astral entity and its level of integration with the incarnate human vehicle of the patient, which leads to inaccurate, ineffective, or inappropriate healing) that allows you to see the way or all of the ways in which an astral entity can attach itself to the incarnate human vehicle.

## The Appearance of an Astral Entity Attached to an Auric Layer

Astral entities can at times choose to attach themselves to the auric layers of the incarnate human vehicle in preference to the energetic templates.

The auric layers are radiation created as a byproduct of the use of the seven main frequencies associated with the incarnate human vehicle as they are assimilated by the chakras and subsequently distributed throughout the incarnate human vehicle. These energies are used to maintain the energy templates that allow the incarnate Aspect to exist within and animate the incarnate human vehicle while maintaining its presence in the lowest frequencies associated with the multiverse, the gross physical aspect of the physical universe. The auric layers can be classified as the "human energy field/s" and are described as such by Barbara Brennan in her books *Hands of Light* and *Light Emerging*.

As a byproduct they can be considered as the "lossy" function, the waste product of the metabolization of these seven frequencies by the chakras.

The auric layers do have a use, however. They provide natural protection from low-grade energetic intrusions and attacks. They can also be augmented and programmed to create an effective and efficient psychic shield for higher grade intrusions and attacks. And, from the perspective of the astral entity, they are a source of free energy.

As an energy field, the auric layers have an electromagnetic function. Each function is specific to the frequency that it is generated on. It is the electromagnetic function of the auric layers that can be used as a coupling device for the incarnate Aspect to connect with other incarnate Aspects who are liked, preferred, loved, trusted, etc. It can also be used as a de-coupling device, repelling those who are not liked, hated, not trusted, we are wary of, etc.

We know that electromagnetic energy can propel

or provide energy or power for electric devices such as motors and electrical/electronic components within a circuit, and astral entities know this as well. It can also be used for attractivity in the form of electromagnets. It is the use of high frequency (above the third frequency) and more subtle levels of electromagnetism that astral entities use to connect with the auric layers of the incarnate human vehicle and take power or energy from. It needs to be noted here that the type of electromagnetism that incarnate mankind uses is very raw and low in frequency relative to that generated as a byproduct by the chakras when metabolizing the frequencies necessary to perpetuate the incarnate human vehicle. Based upon this, no comparison can be made to date with that which science knows as electromagnetism and that which is generated within the functions of the incarnate human vehicle. That said, when it is detected and captured, these frequencies of electromagnetism will open the doors to whole new generations of electronic technologies.

Getting back to astral entities then!

Astral entities use these subtler forms of electromagnetism to link into the auric layers and take energy from them as they are refreshed. Auric layers are refreshed on a continual basis as a function of their being a natural byproduct of the function of the chakras. They are therefore only ever in a position of being un-refreshed when a chakra is functioning in an inefficient way or when the incarnate human vehicle is in the process of demise or has demised. The only other way in which the auric layers are compromised is when an astral entity attaches itself to the layers for energy or the integrity of the overall coverage of an auric layer is diminished leaving a hole when an astral entity moves onto another host, or it is removed and the auric layer is not repaired by the healer who removes the astral entity (see the next section below).

The field of energy and its subtle electromagnetic content effectively creates a slow and almost unperceivable spherical flow of energy in an omnidirectional way around the incarnate human vehicle that can be connected to by the astral entity by using itself as a natural junction, or connection, thereby interrupting the flow for its own purposes. In this way, the astral entity becomes a part of the function of the auric layer or layers that it is connected to, which results in it not being detected by the host. This means that the flow of energy remains but that its power diminishes slightly as it passes around the energy that is the astral entity itself. It is this flow around the astral entity that it uses to sustain its own energy reserves.

Try to think of how this works as when a large boulder interrupts the flow of water in a river, making it go over and around it, locally slowing the passage of water down because it is traveling farther than the water that misses the boulder. It is this additional "distance" that the flow of energy in the auric layer is traveling that the astral entity uses to feed itself.

The healer can only perceive the astral entity as a lump in the normal shape of the auric layer or layers. It is only when the healer uses his/her perception to look at the auric layers in "cross section" that he/she can see that the astral entity is attached in this way to more than one auric layer. It does have to be noted here, though, that the astral entity, using this method, is generally only attached to the auric layers of the seventh, or seventh and sixth frequencies combined. It is rare that the entity selects the energies from the fifth or even the fourth even though they do have to pass through "all" of the auric layers to take energy from the energetic templates.

When the astral entity is embedded into the auric layers in this way, the healer has to be careful how he/she extracts the entity. This is because the removal of the astral entity can cause more problems in terms of maintaining the integrity of the auric layers affected by the entity than by leaving it alone. Basically put, the healer can cause more damage than the entity if he/she does not remove the entity properly and if in removing the entity he/she damages the auric layers and does not repair them.

The process to remove an astral entity from one or more of the auric layers is similar to that used in removing an astral entity from one or more energetic templates. Remember, though, that the energetic templates affect the gross physical aspect of the incarnate human vehicle whereas the auric layers are a byproduct of the chakras that can and are used as a form of protective shield.

"If the auric layers are a byproduct, why do they need to be repaired?" Well, as stated above, the layers are used by us as a form of shield. They are also used as a means of communication between incarnate humans transmitting and receiving emotional responses and personal space advice to those around us. Additionally, if we leave the astral entity within the auric layers, there is a certain level of weight associated with it, which can and does affect the way in which the incarnate human vehicle is animated by the Aspect.

To remove the astral entity from one of the auric layers, the healer must first scan the patient on all seven frequency levels (by opening his/her own chakras) in order to establish which layer/s the entity is occupying. Remember, it is only likely to be one or two layers, and the layers will be from the fourth to the seventh, usually being the sixth and seventh. The astral entity may appear to look similar to, but not the same as, a fish trapped in a fishing net, although the astral entity placed itself there and is not caught in the auric layer per se.

## How to Remove an Astral Entity

Working on the lowest level that you find the astral entity first, gradually use your energetic hands to unravel the entity from the energy of the auric layer. Tease it out. Do your best to remove the entity without damaging the natural matrix or pattern that the auric layer creates as a function of natural radiation. When you have removed the entity from the first layer you may see two entities, one that represents the entity that you have removed from the first layer and another that represents the part of the entity that is still embedded in the higher frequency layer. In this instance, remove the aspect of the entity from the first layer using the method just described, and then place the entity in your recycling bin so that the energy and frequencies of the entity can be reabsorbed into The Source. Don't repair the auric layer until you have removed the entity from all of the levels it has embedded itself into.

Elevate your frequencies to the next level that the entity is on and gently unravel or tease out the entity from the matrix-like structure of that auric layer and place it into your recycling bin. The energies of the entities are now reabsorbed back into the overall energies of The Source.

Now that you have removed the entity, the patient will feel that he/she is balanced and is not carrying around something that he/she can't put his/her finger on. Also, now that you have removed the entity, you can repair any damage to the auric layer/s that the entity may have created, or that was done as a result of the methods used to remove the entity by you as the healer.

As with the method of repairing one of the energetic templates earlier described, the healer should consider the way to repair the auric layer/s in the same way as repairing a fishing net or darning a sock or woollen jumper, criss-crossing the energy lines from north to south and east to west in a weave-based pattern. Once the auric layers have been repaired, the patient may report feeling safer somehow or that a feeling of weakness has gone. He/she may even report feeling whole.

## Holes in the Auric Layers

Holes in the auric layers are usually created by astral entities, either by the way in which they embed themselves within the energy of the layer or through how they take energy from it. The holes can also be created by the astral entity burrowing their way through to the energetic templates.

Such holes are repaired in the way described above.

## Energy Hooks

Another way in which holes can be created in the auric layers is through aggressive or adversarial contact with another incarnate. These holes are created as a function of direct or indirect energetic attack, coercive or controlling energy hooks. They can also be hooks used to allow another incarnate human to feed off another incarnate human's energies. The controlling, feeding, and coercive energy hooks can create a lot of damage if removed in the wrong way by a healer. However, the most damage is caused when the hooks are ripped out by the incarnate Aspect that projected/cast them, or the individual whose auric layer that they are embedded within tears or pulls himself/herself away from the incarnate who projected/ cast them. This is usually done in a desperate attempt to get away from the individual who projected or cast the hooks in the first place.

In the event that energy hooks are found within the auric layers of your patient, as well as removing them in an efficient way, you must trace them back to the individual who projected or cast them in the first place. This is because there may be other links involved such as karmic or past life links between the patient and the individual who projected or cast the hooks that need to be removed as well.

Removing energy hooks can be a delicate process, and although, for those of you who have removed barbed hooks from a fish when going fishing, it may be understood theoretically, much care is required as the hooks created by an adversarial incarnate human can be complicated.

The hooks created by an incarnate human can be multifrequential and multibarbed with many forms of designs or shapes, and removal by simply pulling them can create a lot of damage. The healer will need to access the hook first by elevating their frequencies (by opening the chakras), isolating the frequential position of the lowest auric layer of penetration. The healer then needs to note that all other layers above this level will also be hooked in some way.

For example, if the energy hook penetrates to the third auric layer then the first and second layers will be unaffected, although the third through to the seventh will be affected. In the eventuality that the hook penetrates down to the first layer, then all layers will be affected. If the hook only penetrates to the seventh layer, then only the seventh layer is affected, the sixth through to the first are not. It is also possible that an energy hook may even penetrate the energetic templates as well. In this instance, the healer must consider the energy templates penetrated as additional levels to deal with, potentially creating up to fourteen layers to work with. The added complication here is that the healer will need to work on, for example, the third energy template through to the seventh energy template as well as the first through to the seventh auric layer! If, as in this example this is the case, the healer will need to ensure that he/she makes enough time for the patient so that a hook of this complexity can be removed in one appointment. The healer will also need to have higher than the usual levels of concentration.

Energy hooks can range from the simple, such as a hook with no barb, to those that are very complicated. Such examples may be many hooks on one level or many hooks on each level to levels with every hook in a different location on the hook. This makes removal of the hook a challenge to the healer. However, the auric layers have some inherent functions that can help the healer who is endeavoring to remove a complicated energy hook insomuch as they have a level of pliability or elasticity.

## Removal of a Simple Energy Hook

Having first scanned the patient on all seven levels and establishing that the energy hook is a simple "one-barbed" hook (an even simpler hook would be one that has no barb but that is "J" shaped) that has penetrated the auric layer to the fifth auric layer, for example, the healer needs to start at the lowest frequency. After raising your frequency to that of the fifth frequency level, use your energetic hands to slowly twist and turn the hook to move it away from the fifth auric layer but not so close to the fourth auric layer that you create an additional tear. Then open the tear in the fifth layer and push the hook and barb through the opened tear.

Next, you need to repair the tear in the fifth auric layer and raise your level to the sixth frequency level. Open up the tear in the sixth auric layer and pull the hook through, ensuring that the barb does not create a tear in the newly repaired fifth layer and does not increase the tear in the sixth layer as you pull it through.

Now repair the tear in the sixth auric layer and raise your level to the seventh frequency level. Open up the tear in the seventh auric layer and pull the hook through, ensuring that the barb does not create a tear in the newly repaired sixth layer and does not increase the tear in the seventh layer as you pull it through. Finally, repair the tear in the seventh auric layer and close your chakras so that you descend back to the Earth level of frequency.

Discard the energy hook in the recycling bin that sends the energy to be recycled by The Source (previously mentioned and a normal requirement in energy healing) that your Guide and Helpers have provided for you. This work is now complete, and other healing if required can be concentrated on.

## Illustrations of Energy Hooks

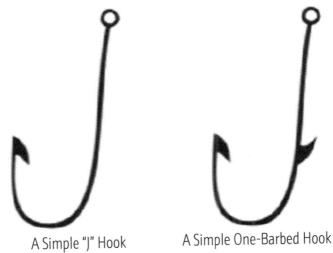

A Simple "J" Hook

A Simple One-Barbed Hook

### Removal of a Complicated Energy Hook

A complicated energy hook is one that has penetrated a number of levels and that has barbs that are effective on all of the levels that the hook has penetrated. This is a particularly difficult operation to undertake and is one that requires an advanced and knowledgeable healer to remove.

In this instance, the healer needs to be able to work on all levels affected at the same time, working in a pan-frequential way. For example, the healer needs to be able to twist and turn the hook and its barbs in such a way that they are able to move the hook further up the auric layers while not creating more damage. It is rather like undoing a combination lock where the combination is the key itself. Based upon this, the healer needs to be able to see the hook on all of the levels penetrated as well as the separate auric layers themselves in a sectioned "sideways" view.

## Illustrations of a Complicated Energy Hook

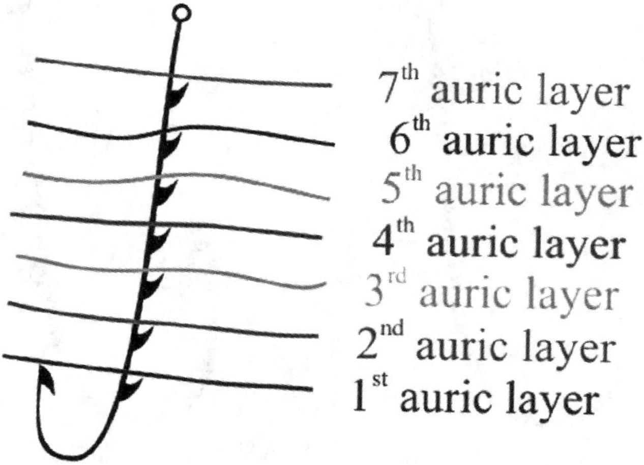


Using the example where the hook has penetrated all seven levels, in order to remove such a hook, the healer, while having all seven chakras open and focusing on being able to be on all levels at once and separately, needs to observe the location of the barbs in relation to each other and the tears in the auric layer that they have made. Remembering that the auric layers have a level of elasticity to them will benefit the healer because sometimes the hooks on the levels do not correlate well with the tears created.

While observing the hook in relation to the tear made in the first auric layer together with checking how the barb of the hook relates to the tears on the second through to the seventh, gently turn and pull the hook so that it aligns with the tear in the first auric layer and if possible, other barbs on other auric layers concurrently. Locally distort the first auric layer close to the first barb extending the tear down over the barb and ease the hook out toward the seventh auric layer. Rotate the hook so that it cannot re-penetrate the first auric layer. While this is being processed, the healer should look to see if any other barbs on the hook can be moved through the second to the seventh auric layers at the same time. If this can be achieved, it is likely that the local distortion or stretching of the auric layer to allow additional extraction is possible. Next, you need to repair the tear in the first auric layer and check to see that you have not created additional tears in the process. If any other barbs were able to be passed through other auric layers, check to see if they can also be repaired or whether they need to be left in place to allow further movement when removing the barbed hook.

Now move on to the second auric layer.

While observing the hook in relation to the tear made in the second auric layer together with checking how the barb of the hook relates to the tears on the third through to the seventh, gently turn and pull the hook so that it aligns with the tear in the second auric layer and if possible, other barbs on other auric layers concurrently. Locally distort the second auric layer close to the first barb extending the tear down over the barb and ease the hook out toward the seventh auric layer. Rotate the hook so that it cannot re-penetrate the second auric layer. While this is being processed, the healer should look to see if any other barbs on the hook can be moved through the third through to the seventh auric layer at the same time. If this can be achieved, it is likely that the local distortion or stretching of the auric layer to allow additional extraction is possible. Next, you need to repair the tear in the second auric layer and check to see that you have not created additional tears in the process. If any other barbs were able to be passed through other auric layers, check to see if they can also be repaired or whether they need to be left in place to allow further movement when removing the barbed hook.

Now move on to the third auric layer.

While observing the hook in relation to the tear made in the third auric layer together with checking how the barb of the hook relates to the tears on the fourth through to the seventh, gently turn and pull the hook so that it aligns with the tear in the third auric layer and if possible, other barbs on other auric layers concurrently. Locally distort the third auric layer close to the first barb extending the tear down over the barb and ease the hook out toward the seventh auric layer. Rotate the hook so that it cannot re-penetrate the third auric layer. While this is being processed, the healer should look to see if any other barbs on the hook can be moved through the fourth through to the seventh auric layer at the same time. If this can be achieved, it is likely that the local distortion or stretching of the auric layer to allow additional extraction is possible. Next, you need to repair the tear in the third auric layer and check to see that you have not created additional tears in the process. If any other barbs were able to be passed through other auric layers, check to see if they can also be repaired or whether they need to be left in place to allow further movement when removing the barbed hook.

Repeat this process for the remaining four auric layers, paying particular attention to the position of the barbs on the hook and their position in relation to the tears and the complicated combination in movement that is required to extract the multibarbed hook through all the tears that have been created while not creating more tears.

It does have to be noted that the level of complication of an energy hook is an indicator of the level of desire that the adversary wishes to inflict in terms of control or pain to or on their prey. As a result of this, it is good practice for the healer to double check for any karmic or past life links with the assailant involved.

Repairing holes or tears in the auric layer

(including the energetic templates) that have been created by adversarial contact with another incarnate human is the same as previously described, that being and in the case of the energetic templates, it is similar to repairing a fishing net with the net being made of energy lines. In the case of the auric layer, it is similar but because the energy auric layers are a byproduct of the energy conversion from the chakras to the energy system at each frequency level, they may be more amorphous. This is achieved in a logical progression with the healer repairing the auric layer that is the lowest frequency first and then moving up the frequencies, affecting repairs layer by layer.

# Astral Mucus Clearing

Astral mucus is low frequency energy that either naturally collects on the outer auric layer, the seventh auric layer as a clump, or is deposited there by an adversarial incarnate individual. It can also be an astral entity of low intelligence, such as that of an amoeba. Indeed, it is more often than not that they look like an amoeba!

Astra mucus therefore tends to resemble an edible jelly that has no form other than that which it adopts if it sets while flat on the ground.

If the astral mucus has not seeped through into the seventh auric layer and onto the sixth, then once the healer has elevated him/herself to the seventh frequency level, it can be peeled off like a lump of jelly or even silicone on a plate. This is relatively simple and very successful if the astral mucus has not seeped into the structure of the auric layer, in which case, it needs to be treated slightly differently. The healer simply has to use their energetic hands to do the peeling. When removed, the astral mucus should be deposited into the ever-useful recycling bin for The Source to reabsorb and reuse the energy. In the event that the astral mucus has indeed seeped into the structure of a single auric layer, then the method of removing the astral mucus from two astral layers illustrated below should also be used for the single layer.

## Illustrations of a Basic Astral Entity (Astral Mucus) Attached to the Other Auric Layers

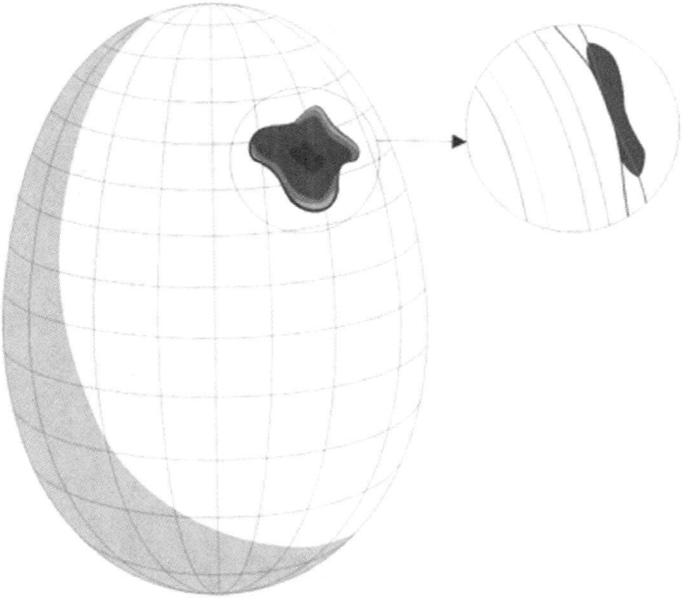

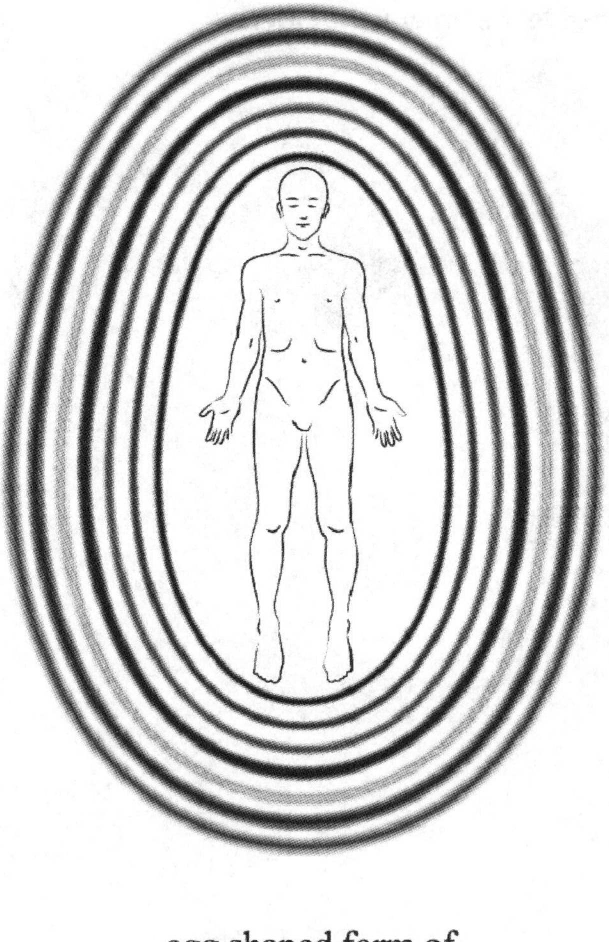

egg shaped form of
auric layers around the human body
(layers are shown in cross section)

The cross-section through all seven auric layers shows the astral mucus seeping through from the 7th onto the 6th auric layer, thus gluing them together.

As stated above, although astral mucus tends to collect on the outer layer of the human aura, the seventh layer, it can often seep into the next layer, the sixth layer. In this instance, the appearance of the auric layers is a bit like having two pieces of tablecloth close together with the auric mucus represented by newly made jelly, that hasn't set that is allowed to seep into the weave of both pieces of tablecloth before eventually setting and subsequently adhering the two pieces of tablecloth together as a jelly-based glue.

In this instance of the jelly with the two pieces of tablecloth, the only way in which the jelly can be removed from the pieces of tablecloth is by washing them in boiling water. The boiling water melts the jelly and dissolves it, allowing the tablecloths to become unattached and clean again.

This illustration shows us that we can achieve the same thing with the astral mucus by increasing the frequency of the auric layer in the locale of the astral mucus. In order to do this, the healer must first elevate him/herself to the seventh frequency and then focus on the location of the astral mucus, sending high frequency energy via the spiritual or third eye to the area of the auric layer where the astral mucus is present.

I can hear you saying now, "I thought that the seventh frequency is the highest frequency that a healer can elevate him/herself to when performing a healing." Well, yes and no. The seventh frequency is the highest level that one can achieve with the use of opening the chakras alone, but it is not the highest frequency that can be achieved by the use of the intention. There are three more frequencies attributed to the incarnate human vehicle's construction. These three higher frequencies are the step-down function that allows the higher frequency energy that is the True Energetic Self to project a small aspect of itself, what we call the soul, into the lowest frequencies of the multiverse, the physical universe, to experience, learn, and evolve through exposure to low frequency existence via an intermediary body—the incarnate human vehicle.

As a result, the healer can invoke the use of these three higher frequencies that are associated with the incarnate human vehicle to assist in the healing process. In this case, the use is required to dissolve a collection of astral mucus that has either permeated the seventh auric layer or both the seventh and the sixth layers together.

Use your intention to visualize that the area occupied (on one or both layers) by the astral mucus is occupied by energy and frequency from the eighth frequency level. See how it starts to make the astral mucus softer, more fluid. If you wish, ask for your Guide and Helpers, or any other healing entities that you work with to create a way to catch the dissolving mucus before it dissolves fully. This can be in the form of an energetic vacuum cleaner, for example. You can also visualize this very useful tool yourself. The vacuum cleaner will perform the same duty as the recycling bin used in other healing processes.

The reason for the use of the vacuum cleaner is because there is a time in the process of dissolving the astral mucus when it is more fluid than viscous and as a result could migrate to the lower frequency auric layers if not removed. In fact, this period between being viscous, fluidic, and totally dissolved is a function of the level of intention of the healer and as such the vacuum cleaner may not be necessary. If the healer is focused, the astral mucus can be dissolved without the intermediate level of becoming fluid, negating the need for the vacuum cleaner.

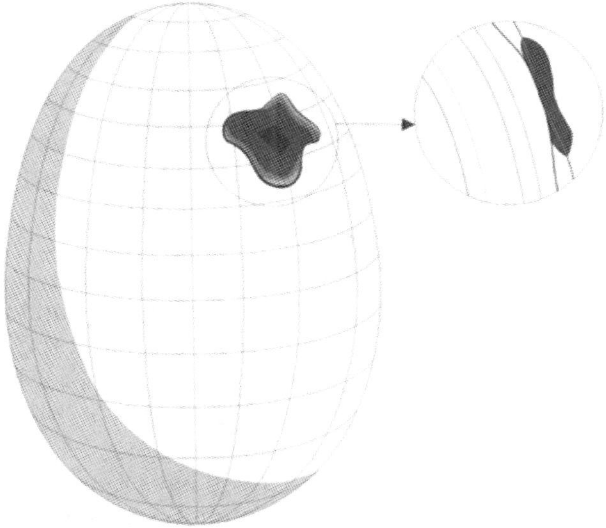

Astral Mucus can be peeled off from the outer seventh auric layer and disposed of in the recycling bin. This is only possible when it hasn't seeped into the sixth layer.

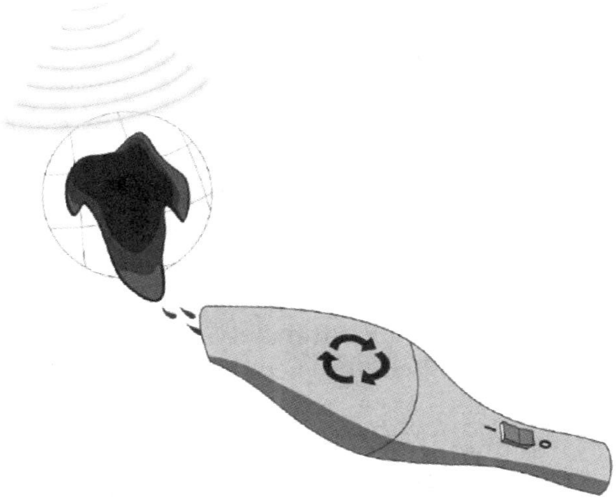

Visualizing a Vacuum Cleaner to Remove the Astral Mucus

However, in the event that the healer does require the vacuum cleaner, it should be ready to use before the astral mucus is dissolved.

As the astral mucus starts to change its state, use the energetic vacuum cleaner to clear out the mucus which moves away from its viscous location as a function of becoming a liquid in form. That which doesn't move will very quickly dissolve and be reabsorbed by The Source in its natural recycling function. Make sure that you are working on the two levels affected concurrently and zoom in with your perceptual vision to check to see if the astral mucus has been removed from both auric layers before you remove your intention on using the energy from the eighth frequency level.

When you are satisfied that you have removed all of the astral mucus, withdraw your intention from the eighth frequency level. Double check that the auric layer/s affected are now clean and clear of any residual astral mucus. If there is residual mucus, the whole process must be repeated as astral mucus attracts astral mucus very effectively.

Now scan all seven of the auric layers and notice how resplendent this energetic byproduct of the chakras receiving seven frequency levels of energy to animate the incarnate human form appears. If you don't see the aura, the human energy field, as resplendent, then you need to check to see what else needs to be healed or repaired.

I suggest that this is the best process to use when the healer observes astral mucus that has pervaded one or more auric layers. Trying to energetically pull or scrape the astral mucus away from the auric layer/s will create more work as you will ultimately tear the auric layer concerned and will therefore need to repair the auric layer as well.

As with all of the healing functions or modalities in this book, patience is a virtue and the healer must allot enough time for the patient to ensure that the healing is complete in one session. Trying to administer this sort of work over two or more sessions is detrimental to the patient because it leaves them in an incomplete state of healing and vulnerable to further attack.

# Crossed Hara Lines (Lines of Projection) with Other Incarnates from the Same or Different True Energetic Self

The Hara Line is the connection between the True Energetic Self (TES) and the incarnate Aspect (soul). It enters the physical universe at the $12^{th}$ frequency and connects to the incarnate human vehicle via the step-down functions supported by the $10^{th}$, $9^{th}$, and $8^{th}$ frequencies. It then moves through to the energetic templates that are associated with the gross physical frequencies of the $1^{st}$, $2^{nd}$, and $3^{rd}$ levels and the spirituo-physical levels of the $4^{th}$, $5^{th}$, $6^{th}$, and $7^{th}$ frequencies. The sentience and energy of the Aspect divide at the Core Star with the sentience moving to the Soul Seat and the energies to animate the incarnate human vehicle moving to the Tan Tien.

The Tan Tien is where the energy of the Aspect spreads out into the energy network that contains the energy template and the chakras. It ends up being a focus of tremendous energy. It is positioned two inches (5 cm) below the navel (belly button) and three inches (7.5 cm) in toward the center of the human vehicle from the navel.

The Soul Seat is where the sentience of the Aspect resides. It is the personality of what we, as a projected Aspect of our TES, are; "it is our sentience." Its position is close to where the front and rear Aspects of the heart chakra join, close to the thymus.

The Core Star is the point or location of the division of sentience and energy of the incarnate Aspect within the human vehicle. The energy used to animate the human vehicle coalesces in the Tan Tien (located two inches below the navel and three inches in toward the center of the body) with the sentience coalescing in the Soul Seat (located close the point where the front and rear aspects of the heart chakras are joined or located, close to the thymus). The Core Star is often mistaken for the Tan Tien as it is so close to the Core Star. The Core Star is positioned two inches (5 cm) above the navel (belly button) and three inches (7.5 cm) in toward the center of the human vehicle from the navel.

## Illustrations of the Hara Lines in Conjunction to the Chakra

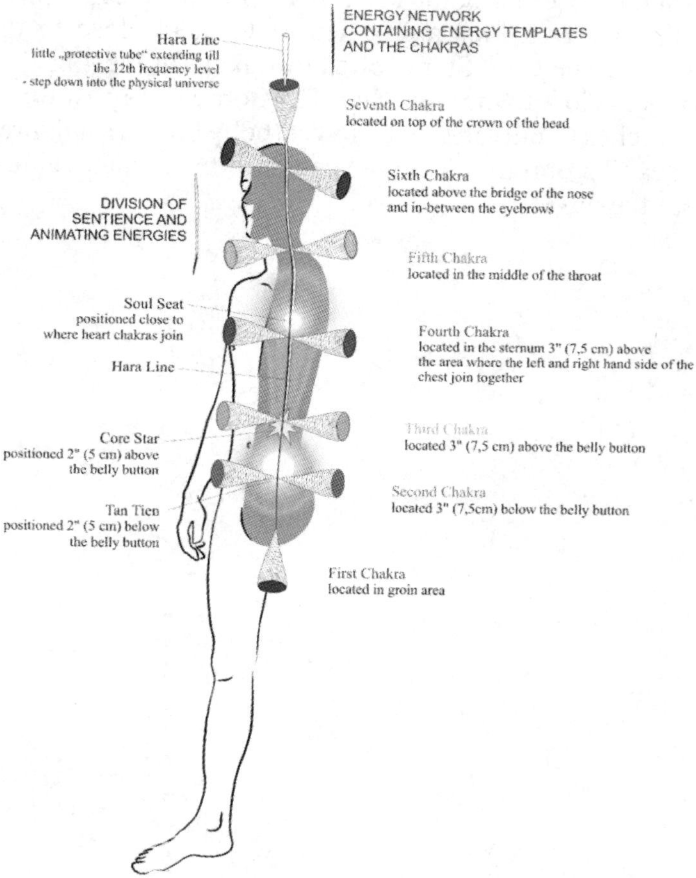
ENERGY NETWORK
CONTAINING ENERGY TEMPLATES
AND THE CHAKRAS
Hara Line
little „protective tube" extending till
the 12th frequency level
- step down into the physical universe
Seventh Chakra
located on top of the crown of the head
Sixth Chakra
located above the bridge of the nose
and in-between the eyebrows
DIVISION OF
SENTIENCE AND
ANIMATING ENERGIES
Fifth Chakra
located in the middle of the throat
Soul Seat
positioned close to
where heart chakras join
Fourth Chakra
located in the sternum 3" (7,5 cm) above
the area where the left and right hand side of the
chest join together
Hara Line
Core Star
positioned 2" (5 cm) above
the belly button
Third Chakra
located 3" (7,5 cm) above the belly button
Second Chakra
located 3" (7,5cm) below the belly button
Tan Tien
positioned 2" (5 cm) below
the belly button
First Chakra
located in groin area

Crossed Hara Lines (Lines of Projection) with Other Incarnates from the Same or Different True Energetic Self

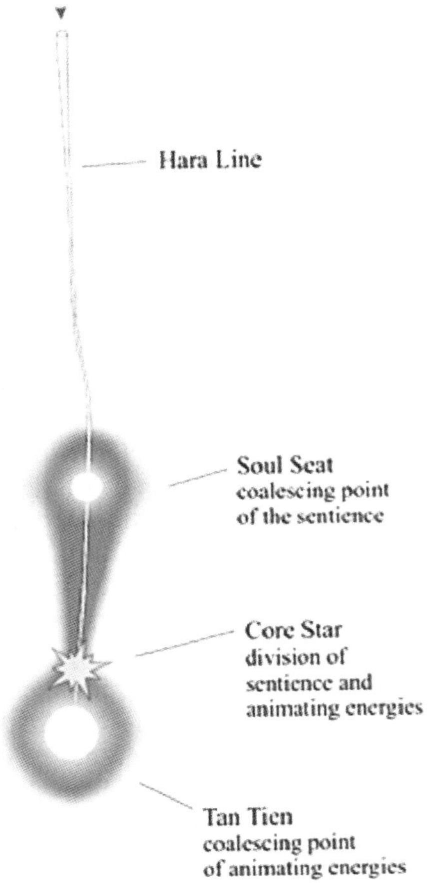


Entanglement is when the energetic or Hara Lines of projection between two or more Aspects occurs. It can occur between Aspects of the same TES or between Aspects of different TES. It may seem bizarre that this can happen at all in an environment where a TES can be a master of its energies and environment, but it does. Especially when the Aspects in question are being projected by TES (*the plural of TES is TES —GSN*) that are close to each other frequentially and environmentally.

Although not an issue in the energetic because we experience a much higher level of individual and shared/ collective connectivity and expansiveness from the perspective of being incarnate, entanglement can and does create issues between the Aspects whose Hara Lines are crossed or entangled, especially in the lowest frequencies of the physical universe and therefore the multiverse. When the lines of projection are crossed or entangled, the communication between the projected Aspect and its TES can be shared by those experiencing entanglement. However, if there is no understanding of the simultaneous experiences that can be achieved by the TES and its Aspects, by the TES, and that all Aspects experiencing entanglement also share these experiences, then when these simultaneous experiences happen, confusion reigns.

The incarnate Aspect, when in the lowest frequencies of the physical universe, generally has no knowledge of the ability of the functions associated with entanglement, and so when they are experiencing the thoughts associated with the experience of imagery, knowledge, and audible data that is invariably divorced from the environment the Aspect is incarnate within, the Aspect loses total association with the primary environment incarnated into. For example, if the Aspect experiencing the simultaneous environments and experiences of another incarnate is based on Earth and the Aspect that it is entangled with is based in another environment in another galaxy, then that audiovisual data has no anchor point to the Earth-based environment the Earth-based incarnate Aspect has, and so it will have no place in the total vocabulary set of this incarnate Aspect.

The total vocabulary set in this instance is not just the spoken language but also the sum of the total experiential content experienced, such as the five physical senses and thoughts, desires, lessons, etc., accrued by the incarnate Aspect. So, the incarnate Aspect experiencing the experiential content of another Aspect either develops a fear of that which it experiences, specifically if it is not of the Earth-based environment or accepts it and openly tries to communicate with that which is experienced by the other Aspect. The ultimate destination for the incarnate Aspect that develops either the fear of or desire to communicate with that which it experiences is psychosis or schizophrenia and the development of mental health issues. The ultimate end-game is usually the administration of a regime of medication and/or sedation.

It is possible, with the correct teaching, to help the incarnate Aspect understand what it is experiencing and work with it in a positive and functional way that does not attract the attention of mental health professionals while maintaining this rare connectivity. However, healing performed correctly can untwine the Hara Lines of the affected Aspects and return them to the normal isolation incarnate Aspects experience.

In summary then, patients who are experiencing detachment from their current reality, observations from another reality, hearing strange voices in a language that is not their own, or even not of the Earth, may also have the feeling that they have lost time or have memories that they cannot attribute to be their own. Having the energetic link, the Hara Line, between them and their TES crossed with the energetic link, the Hara Line of another incarnate aspect from either the same TES or another TES can and does create all these symptoms.

Although the medical reference to this condition may be classified as schizophrenia, there are two metaphysical reasons for the patient being diagnosed in this way, crossed Hara Lines just discussed being one of them. The other is being associated with more than one Aspect or soul in one single incarnate vehicle. I will discuss this and the appropriate healing process in a later chapter.

In order to establish if this is the case, healers need to elevate themselves to the seventh level by opening the chakras and then use their intention to ease their consciousness up the next three frequencies to that of the tenth frequency. From this position, the healer can focus his/her intention to move away from the frequencies of his/her own incarnate vehicle, and the last two frequencies of the physical universe, the eleventh and twelfth, and perceive the Hara Line in its multifrequential condition, that being, to see it represented on all of the frequencies it passes through. When you can perceive it in this way (I personally perceive it as a red line), focus your intention to trace it back to its connectivity with the TES.

As you trace the Hara Line back through the frequencies, you may perceive the Hara Lines of other incarnate Aspects associated with the TES you are tracing this Hara Line back to, or other incarnate Aspects projected from another TES. If while tracing the Hara Line of your patient back to his/her TES, you observe that your patient's Hara Line is entwined with the Hara Line of another Aspect, either of the patient's TES or another unrelated TES, then this creates the possibility of both Aspects receiving the experiences of the other. As stated above, one can imagine this can create all sorts of psychological issues at the human level of perspective. You may perceive an unfocused or fuzzy image of both Aspects as a result of the entwining.

## Untwining the Hara Line

By the same process used to establish that your patient has their Hara Line entwined with the Hara Line of another incarnate Aspect, the healer needs to make full use of his/her focus and intention to perceive the level of entanglement. The Hara Lines can therefore be entwined more than once and so the process of untwining them needs to include multiple untwining operations. It is not likely that a knot is created, and although this may be a possibility, it is so remote that I have never seen such entanglement. We have to give the projected Aspects some credit for navigation while incarnate. It is worth noting that the location and interaction between incarnate Aspects in the physical universe is not indicative of the level of entanglement, or even if entanglement is manifest because it is a function of the movement of the TES and their projected Aspects and how they interact with other TES and Aspects in the energetic that causes this issue.

Using your perception, see the two aspects and their Hara Lines as the same size as a marionette, knowing that you can move the incarnate Aspects around each other with your energetic hands. This means zooming out from them and perceiving them from a distance to give them the perspective of being small and manipulatable.

Take one of the Aspects with your energetic hands and hold it in a static position with your intention, ensuring that it cannot move. This is going to make the untwining easier for you because you will only need to do the actual untwining with one Aspect and its Hara Line. Next, take the other Aspect and slowly move the Aspect in the opposite direction that the entwining was created. For example, if the entwining is clockwise to the other Aspect's position, the untwining must be counterclockwise. Although this is common sense, it is best to perform the untwining in a logical, slow, and careful way because rapid untwining can affect both incarnate Aspects, making them disoriented or even causing them to experience loss of balance. Slowly and methodically untwine the two Aspects and their Hara Lines from each other and when finished, place the Aspects some distance from each other ensuring that the Hara Lines are stretched to a taut condition.

Now move yourself back to the Earth level of frequency and observe the change in your patient. You will see a look of calmness in his/her face and any irritation that he/she may have displayed will not be present. However, although you may see a change in your patient's demeanor, your patient may take a few days to actually notice the difference in him/herself. Although, those that are experiencing constant levels of disorientation will notice the difference quickly, especially if they have been hearing the voices of, or seeing images of, other communications and experiential content of those incarnate Aspects whose Hara Lines they have been entangled with. In essence, their schizophrenia will cease.

Finally, there is a possibility that more than two Aspects have their Hara Line entwined or entangled. However, the process for untwining or unentangling the Hara Line of more than two Aspects is the same, although potentially more complicated, and must be performed at the same time.

# Virus Clearing

Viruses are cell-based infections and they can spread around the body or within an organ at a rapid rate. Virus clearing is only generally required when the patient is experiencing continual levels of infection that are not apparently clearing up. Colds, influenza, and their variants are those viruses that the healer are not likely to be asked to heal as many people accept and work with them. However, other viruses such as those found in organs, for example, the kidneys or the liver, can produce debilitating results for the patient, including and up to organ failure through the creation of disease.

In order to treat a viral infection, the healer first needs to raise his/her frequency to that of the seventh level and perform a full body scan on all seven frequency levels concurrently with the use of their perceptual vision and intuition to establish where the epicenter of the viral outbreak originated from, and more important, where it has spread to.

Because viruses are arguably a microorganism (although there is some debate over this) and therefore have DNA, they will respond to DNA-based reprogramming to change the way in which they function. Viruses proliferate by forcing the cells that they are using as a host to reproduce themselves.

Fortunately for the healer, DNA is and can be programmed by RNA energetically, using the process below, which in turn is used as a biological communication agent between DNA and cell protein. Based upon this, if the healer focuses upon reprogramming the DNA (via the energetic aspect of RNA) of the virus at its epicenter, then that reprogramming will be naturally transmitted throughout the network of affected cells during reproduction and place the opportunity for further reproduction either into stasis or arrest.

DNA reprogramming is ultimately one of the functions of psycho-spiritual reprogramming described later in this book. However, it is worth explaining this part in summary here as it is the best way to heal the patient who has a virus.

While you are scanning the body of the patient, you will need to establish the epicenter of the viral outbreak and the other areas of the body where it has spread to and where it is likely to spread to as a function of the flow of blood and cells.

When you have established where the majority of the virus is (it may even be contained within an organ and has not yet spread to any other part of the body), visualize yourself zooming into the virus and see its structure. Then zoom in further with your mind's eye using it like an electron microscope getting closer and closer to the basic structure of the virus until you see the string of DNA that is the basis of its size, shape, variant, and function. Ask your intuition to point you toward the area of the DNA that controls the reproductive cycle of the virus. Make a note of the area and what that portion of DNA looks like, and how it is linked to the RNA.

Next visualize the RNA and ask to see the energetic aspect of the RNA associated with the reproductive cycle. Visualize the energetics of the RNA as an array of switches, each switch being associated with a function of the virus. You may perceive many functions of the virus such as proliferation rate, cells to be attracted to, ways to infiltrate cells, ways to be disguised, and preferred organs to collect within.

Proliferation rate would be a good switch to work with. However, you may see this as a method of adjustment rather than turning the proliferation on or off.

The adjustment of the proliferation may look like a volume control knob. Irrespective of how you perceive the way to change the proliferation or the rate of reproduction of the virus, you should be able to turn or adjust it right down to zero using your energetic hand to do just that and stop the proliferation of the virus by turning it down to zero. Or, if you are presented with an on/off switch, turn it off.

Once the proliferation of the virus is either turned off or reduced to zero, the virus will start to be affected by the program change that you have set at the energetic level and reprogram the DNA of the virus. Using your perceptual vision, zoom into the DNA again. You will see that the DNA of the virus is being affected and that one of the "rungs" on the DNA ladder is missing from the area that donates the desire for the virus to proliferate. You may also perceive the program from the DNA being sent to the virus and the speed of proliferation of the virus being dramatically reduced as the change in the program takes effect. Now zoom out from observing the DNA of the virus, reduce your frequency level down to the zero level, the Earth level, and look at the demeanor of the patient. You may see an immediate affect and the patient may state that he/she is starting to feel better.

# Spine Cleansing

A patient that has pain in the back at any level, curvature of the spine, or feels that they have an energy blockage may need to have the energy flow of the spine realigned by the use of spine cleansing. The administration of a spine cleanse provides the patient with a profound healing and as such they will need to be given time for "after treatment" respite in a quiet place to recover from the work before returning to his/her daily routine.

The spine cleansing technique is complicated and time-consuming and will need to be performed on each and every vertebra on every one of the seven energetic templates and therefore on every frequency level where they are represented. This means that the healer works on a vertebra injecting energy into it one frequency level at a time from frequency level one through seven before they can move on to the next vertebra. It is a tiring process and as such the spine cleansing technique should only be performed by an experienced healer who has in turn been trained and supervised in the administration of the technique by an experienced and knowledgeable healing instructor. As a result, this chapter should be used for illustrative purposes only and not as an instructional text in how to perform the spine cleansing.

## Preparation

The healer will need to practice moving up and down the frequencies in quick succession first by opening the chakras one by one from the base chakra through to the crown chakra and back down again over a period of two to three minutes to ensure that they are capable of moving at the correct speed and affect the cleansing at the correct frequency level for each vertebra. This takes continuous concentration and as stated above can be, and is, tiring. As such I very much feel that the healer who performs this healing function should only perform one healing, the spine cleansing, on any particular day. As such, the healer needs to plan the appointment for the patient as a result of prior consultation and should not be performed "on the hoof" and in the middle of other appointments, so to speak. Clearly an extremely experienced healer may be able to do this, but it will still result in the healer experiencing tiredness as a result of the level of concentration needed, which is detrimental to their performance and quality of healing for the next patient/s.

The patient will need to wear light clothing over the upper body so that you can feel the vertebrae with your fingers. You may need to loosen trousers or the waistline of a skirt to affect the spine cleansing on the lower lumbar region.

## One Vertebra at a Time

There are thirty-three bones in the human spine. Seven vertebrae in the cervical region, twelve in the thoracic region, five in the lumbar region, five in the sacral region, and four in the coccygeal region. The cervical (neck) are classified as C1–C7, the thoracic (main back) are classified as T1–T12, the lumbar (lower back) are classified as L1–L5, and the sacral are classified as S1–S5. The coccygeal are not normally classified separately and are sometimes referred to simply as the coccyx. However, for the performance of the spine cleansing, we will progress from L5, the bottom lumbar vertebra, through the thoracic vertebrae to C1 of the cervical vertebrae, the top of the neck. This is because the sacral and coccygeal (coccyx) vertebrae are too small to affect a hands-on healing. They will be addressed as a function of the overall spine in the final part of the spine cleansing process classified as an energy flush and movement activation process.

## Illustration of the Human Spine

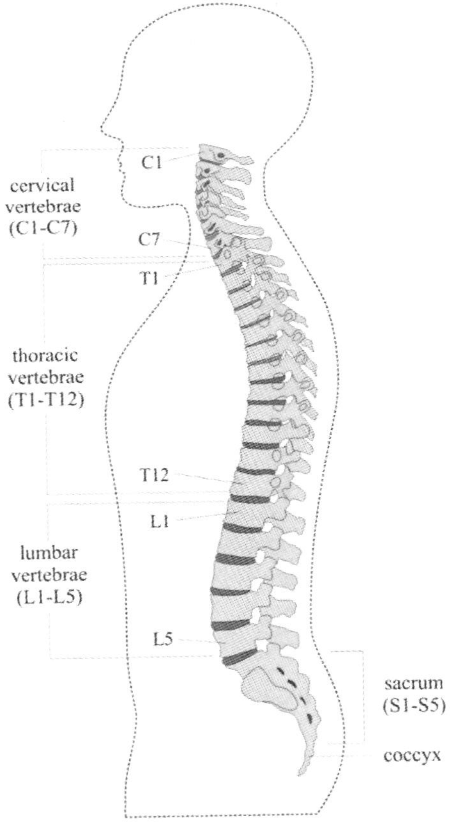


left lateral view

To perform the spine cleansing, ask the patient to lie face down on your therapy bed (ensuring that the head is well supported and that the patient can breathe without strain) with the head to your left and the feet to your right.

Open your first or base chakra and elevate your frequency to the first level. Place the forefinger and thumb of your right hand on the lower aspect of L5 (where it meets S1 of the sacral vertebra) and the forefinger and thumb of your left hand on the upper aspect of L5 (where it meets L4 of the lumbar vertebrae). Now visualize (or use a mentally spoken command) that you are injecting first frequency energy from the lower aspect of L5 to the upper aspect of L5. Use your visualization or your intuition to feel when the vertebra you are working on has absorbed the level of first frequency energy that it needs.

## Illustration of Placing the Forefinger and Thumb on a Vertebra

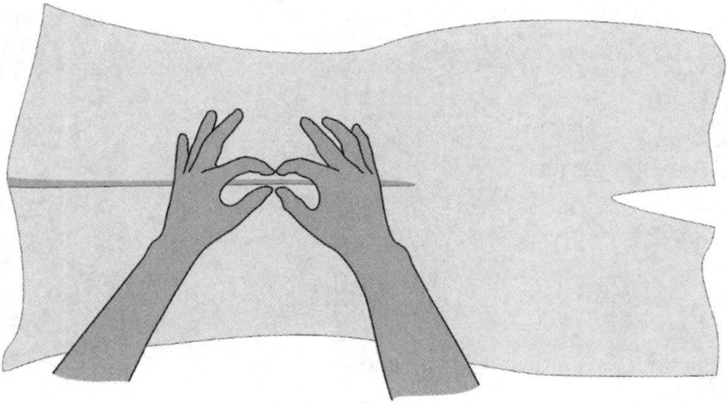

Now open your sacral chakra to elevate you to the second frequency level and inject second frequency energy from the lower aspect of L5 to the upper aspect of L5. Use your visualization or your intuition to feel when the vertebra you are working on has absorbed the level of second frequency energy that it needs.

Open your solar chakra to elevate you to the third frequency level and inject third frequency energy from the lower aspect of L5 to the upper aspect of L5. Use your visualization or your intuition to feel when the vertebra you are working on has absorbed the level of third frequency energy that it needs.

Open your heart chakra to elevate you to the fourth frequency level and inject fourth frequency energy from the lower aspect of L5 to the upper aspect of L5. Use your visualization or your intuition to feel when the vertebra you are working on has absorbed the level of fourth frequency energy that it needs.

Open your throat chakra to elevate you to the fifth frequency level and inject fifth frequency energy from the lower aspect of L5 to the upper aspect of L5. Use your visualization or your intuition to feel when the vertebra you are working on has absorbed the level of fifth frequency energy that it needs.

Open your spiritual or third eye chakra to elevate you to the sixth frequency level and inject sixth frequency energy from the lower aspect of L5 to the upper aspect of L5. Use your visualization or your intuition to feel when the vertebra you are working on has absorbed the level of sixth frequency energy that it needs.

Finally open your crown chakra to elevate you to the seventh frequency level and inject seventh frequency energy from the lower aspect of L5 to the upper aspect of L5. Use your visualization or your intuition to feel when the vertebra you are working on has absorbed the level of seventh frequency energy that it needs.

Once you have injected energy from all seven levels into vertebra L5 close chakras seven through one, one by one, and move your hands on to the next vertebra, L4.

Open your base or root chakra to elevate your frequencies to that of the first frequency level. Place the forefinger and thumb of your right hand on the lower aspect of L4 (where it meets L5 of the lumbar vertebrae) and the forefinger and thumb of your left hand on the upper aspect of L4 (where it meets L3 of the lumbar vertebrae). Now visualize (or use a mentally spoken command) that you are injecting first frequency energy from the lower aspect of L4 to the upper aspect of L4. Use your visualization or your intuition to feel when the vertebra you are working on has absorbed the level of first frequency energy that it needs.

Continue in the same fashion on L4 as you did on L5, working your way up the frequencies by opening your chakras one by one and injecting energy into the vertebra frequency level by frequency level. Don't forget to close your chakras one by one to bring you down to the zero or Earth frequency level before you move onto the next vertebra.

Now use this process to work your way up the vertebrae one by one, injecting energy into the vertebrae frequency level by frequency level, finally finishing at vertebra C1.

To finish, close your chakras one by one from the crown through to the base or root chakra to return back to the zero or Earth frequency level.

## Overall Spine Cleanse

Once the vertebrae have been individually cleansed on all seven levels, the healer can elect to perform an additional cleanse to all vertebrae concurrently (at the same time). The process below is identical to the individual vertebra but incorporates all of the vertebrae.

Open your first or base chakra and elevate your frequency to the first level. Place the forefinger and thumb of your right hand on the lower aspect of L5 (where it meets S1 of the sacral vertebra) and the forefinger and thumb of your left hand on the upper aspect of C1 (where it meets the bottom of the skull). Now visualize (or use a mentally spoken command) that you are injecting first frequency energy from the lower aspect of L5 to the upper aspect of C1. Use your visualization or your intuition to feel when the vertebrae have absorbed the level of first frequency energy that they need.

Now open your sacral chakra to elevate you to the second frequency level and inject second frequency energy from the lower aspect of L5 to the upper aspect of C1. Use your visualization or your intuition to feel when the vertebrae have absorbed the level of second frequency energy that they need.

Open your solar chakra to elevate you to the third

frequency level and inject third frequency energy from the lower aspect of L5 to the upper aspect of C1. Use your visualization or your intuition to feel when the vertebrae have absorbed the level of third frequency energy that they need.

Open your heart chakra to elevate you to the fourth frequency level and inject fourth frequency energy from the lower aspect of L5 to the upper aspect of C1. Use your visualization or your intuition to feel when the vertebrae have absorbed the level of fourth frequency energy that they need.

Open your throat chakra to elevate you to the fifth frequency level and inject fifth frequency energy from the lower aspect of L5 to the upper aspect of C1. Use your visualization or your intuition to feel when the vertebrae have absorbed the level of fifth frequency energy that they need.

Open your spiritual or third eye chakra to elevate you to the sixth frequency level and inject sixth frequency energy from the lower aspect of L5 to the upper aspect of C1. Use your visualization or your intuition to feel when the vertebrae have absorbed the level of sixth frequency energy that they need.

Finally, open your crown chakra to elevate you to the seventh frequency level and inject seventh frequency energy from the lower aspect of L5 to the upper aspect of C1. Use your visualization or your intuition to feel when the vertebrae have absorbed the level of seventh frequency energy that they need.

Once you have injected energy from all seven levels into vertebra L5 to C1 close your chakras one by one from the crown through to the base or root chakra to return back to the zero or Earth frequency level. Next work on the spinal energy flush.

## Spinal Energy Flush and Energy Flow Activation

The final process is to flush out any excess energies

from the spine starting from the coccyx through to C1. This process also ensures that the energy flow through the spine is activated. Although we have ignored the sacral and coccyx vertebrae in the previous processes as a result of not being able to effectively connect with them from a "hands-on" perspective, we can include them in this process by using our intention.

Position the right hand, palm down, over the coccyx area without making physical contact and then place the left hand on top of the right with the palm of the left hand on the top of the right hand.

Open your base or root chakra to elevate your frequency to the first frequency level. Next rotate your hands in a counterclockwise fashion three times around the area of the coccyx using the coccyx as the center point of the rotation. Once you have finished the third rotation, move the hands up the spine from the coccyx to vertebra C1 in an accelerated way. This moves the first frequency energy up the spine removing any energetic excess and assuring energetic flow on this level.

## Illustration of the Palm on Hand Counterclockwise Rotation

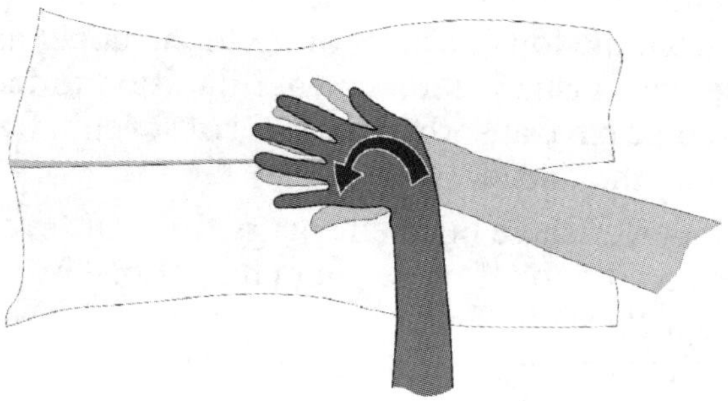

Open your sacral chakra to elevate your frequency to the second frequency level. Rotate your hands in the counterclockwise fashion three times around the area of the coccyx using the coccyx as the center point of the rotation. Once you have finished the third rotation, move the hands up the spine from the coccyx to vertebra C1 in an accelerated way. This moves the second frequency energy up the spine removing any energetic excess and assuring energetic flow on this level.

Open your solar chakra to elevate your frequency to the third frequency level. Rotate your hands in the counterclockwise fashion three times around the area of the coccyx using the coccyx as the center point of the rotation. Once you have finished the third rotation, move the hands up the spine from the coccyx to vertebra C1 in an accelerated way. This moves the third frequency energy up the spine removing any energetic excess and assuring energetic flow on this level.

Open your heart chakra to elevate your frequency to the fourth frequency level. Rotate your hands in the counterclockwise fashion three times around the area of the coccyx using the coccyx as the center point of the rotation. Once you have finished the third rotation, move the hands up the spine from the coccyx to vertebra C1 in an accelerated way. This moves the fourth frequency energy up the spine removing any energetic excess and assuring energetic flow on this level.

Open your throat chakra to elevate your frequency to the fifth frequency level. Rotate your hands in the counterclockwise fashion three times around the area of the coccyx using the coccyx as the center point of the rotation. Once you have finished the third rotation, move the hands up the spine from the coccyx to vertebra C1 in an accelerated way. This moves the fifth frequency energy up the spine removing any energetic excess and assuring energetic flow on this level.

Open your spiritual or third eye chakra to elevate your frequency to the sixth frequency level. Rotate your hands in the counterclockwise fashion three times around the area of the coccyx using the coccyx as the center point of the rotation. Once you have finished the third rotation, move the hands up the spine from the coccyx to vertebra C1 in an accelerated way. This moves the sixth frequency energy up the spine removing any energetic excess and assuring energetic flow on this level.

Finally, open your crown chakra to elevate your frequency to the seventh frequency level. Rotate your hands in the counterclockwise fashion three times around the area of the coccyx using the coccyx as the center point of the rotation. Once you have finished the third rotation, move the hands up the spine from the coccyx to vertebra C1 in an accelerated way. This moves the seventh frequency energy up the spine removing any energetic excess and assuring energetic flow on this level.

Once you have completed this process, close your chakras down one by one until you are on the zero or Earth frequency level.

Ensure both the patient and you rest for a few minutes and drink some water to help ground you both.

Please note that when performing this final process in the spine cleansing that the patient may experience, and the healer will therefore witness, spasms or dramatic energy shifts or movement in the spinal area and upper back. This is a natural and expected response to this very deep level of healing and is nothing to worry about.

Also note that the patient will also feel very disoriented and dizzy. Again, this is a natural and expected response.

# Brain Balancing and Clearing

Brain balancing is a technique that is required when the patient has a problem with seeing and interacting with people and issues surrounding them. They may claim to be seeing through fog or demonstrate an inability to understand even simple things. The patient may claim to be "fuzzy headed," unable to think straight, dizzy, or confused.

When the patient demonstrates the symptoms above, it's clear that they may have one of two things wrong with them energetically. First, the energetic templates associated with the brain can be covered in low frequency energy. This low frequency energy can manifest itself, while covering or infesting the brain, on all seven energetic templates as dust to the perceptual vision of the healer. Second, it can look like smoke or fog in and around the brain and the head itself.

In the event that none of the above manifestations is being perceived by the healer then the energetic functions of the brain may be "out of balance," which can also cause the symptoms identified above.

All of the above can be classified as being "out of focus" or as having a "lack of focus."

## Brain Clearing

Brain clearing is a function of visualization and the use of the visualizations to affect the desire, intention, thought, and action of healing are, by and large, extremely powerful. They also tend to speak to the needs of the patient and the way in which the healer heals the ailment. Because of this, the visualizations discussed in this book are best used by the healer as an example rather than as how "they may" perform the visualization themselves.

Having first established that the reason for the patient's "lack of focus" is due to the brain being covered or infested in low frequency energy, the healer will need to clear this energy on all seven levels of the energy templates—one by one. As previously explained, the healer can elevate their own frequency by opening the chakras one by one to affect the clearing of the low frequency energy from the brain and surrounding area.

The healer should therefore open their own base chakra to elevate themselves to the first frequency level and then visualize the use of a vacuum cleaner to suck up the low frequency energy from the area outside of the brain. This area can be in between the brain and the inside of the skull or outside of the periphery of the head in general. The low frequency energy that infests the brain on this first level, and subsequent levels, can be cleared by visualizing the energetic template of the brain as a hologram giving the healer the ability to move the suction nozzle of the vacuum cleaner in and out of the image of the brain.

Once you have cleaned or cleared the low frequency energy from either inside or outside the brain, or indeed both, you can move on to the second frequency level by opening your sacral chakra. Repeat the work you did on the first level on this second frequency level, then by opening the chakras one by one, the remaining levels. When you have cleaned and cleared the low frequency energy from the seventh level, close each chakra, again one by one, until you are back on the zero or Earth level.

It is possible that the experienced healer may be able to affect a brain cleansing/clearing on all seven levels concurrently. However, if you have not performed this technique before, it is best to clean/clear each level one by one, level by level, on a number of patients until you are fully conversant with the process and feel that you can affect a healing on all seven levels (visualizing all seven levels concurrently with all seven chakras open) without loss of effectivity of the depth of clearing/cleansing.

To check the effectivity of the brain cleansing, ask the patient a few random questions about either themselves or a publicly known subject and observe how fast, coherent, knowledgeable they respond. The clarity of response in terms of understanding and responding to the questions will advise you of the effectivity of the cleaning/clearing preformed. In the event that the client instantly feels an improvement in the way in which they can think then the process of further healing via brain balancing will not be necessary. However, if the patient is still demonstrating a lower level of focus, even though it may be an improvement over that which they demonstrated when first entering your therapy room then they will benefit from brain balancing.

## Brain Balancing

Whereas the brain clearing/cleansing is performed frequency level by frequency level, the brain (energy) balancing technique is performed without reference to any particular level. In this instance, it is simply the intention of the healer to balance the energies of the brain that is required.

However, although it is only the intention of the healer that is required to balance the energies of the brain, physical or near physical contact of the palms of the hands with the left and right temples of the head are also necessary.

As most healers and spiritual individuals are aware, the palms of the hands are the location of two of the minor chakras associated with the human energy system. They are particularly useful when actively directing energy to a certain location.

To perform brain balancing the healer simply needs to place the palms of the hands on the temples of the head of the patient and then ask, with their mentally spoken words, for the balancing energies to flow through their hands into the brain of the patient. This is best achieved by the healer being behind the patient so that the healer's right palm is on the patient's right temple with the left palm on the left temple. The healer (and the patient) may then feel the balancing energies flowing from one palm to the other and back again. It may even feel like the energy is circular (circulating) or oscillating. When this feeling of "moving energy" subsides the brain balancing is completed, and the healer can remove their hands from the temples of the head of the patient.

Again, check how clear the patient's thinking is with the same method explained above.

Although brain balancing and brain clearing/cleansing can be performed in isolation to each other it is best to check the results of these modalities of healing to see if further balancing or cleansing/clearing is required or would be of benefit to the patient from a supplementary perspective.

# Hara Line Healing / Realignment

The Hara Line is the medium in which the True Energetic Self (TES) is able to project a smaller aspect of its sentience and energy (what we sometimes call the Soul) in to a lower frequency environment while maintaining operational connectivity with that smaller aspect.

The Hara Line has many functions that can be classified as psycho-spiritual or intentional in nature. That being, our intention or reason to be, our life purpose or plan! One can therefore argue that the intention of the TES to project a smaller aspect of itself into the lowest frequencies of the multiverse to experience, learn, and evolve does, in itself, create the intention for the Hara to be in existence in its own right. With the Hara Line in existence, we as incarnate entities, therefore have the means to have the intention to be "in existence" in the lowest frequencies of the multiverse.

Many healers focus on the psycho-spiritual side of the function of the Hara Line in terms of realignment of the life (incarnation) purpose or plan as a means of realigning the Hara Line. This is also classified as healing the Hara Line. Indeed, most of the energetic functions and organs associated with the incarnate human vehicle have a psycho-spiritual aspect to them. For instance, the front aspect of the five groups of horizontal chakras, the sacral chakra to the spiritual or third eye chakra, are psycho-spiritually associated with our intention, whereas the rear aspect of these chakras, psycho-spiritually, is our action. However, psycho-spiritual healing is, by and large, intangible and difficult to understand and as such is the ability to heal the patient psycho-spiritually in a robust and repeatable way. This means that realignment of the Hara Line from the perspective of the life purpose or intention needs to be healed purely from a psycho-spiritual perspective. Also, the Hara Line may not even be associated with any psycho-spiritual healing that is required to heal the patient's intention, life purpose, or focus!

However, the Hara Line, if damaged energetically, needs another method of healing. Based upon this, I will be dealing with psycho-spiritual healing in a later chapter and deal with my understanding of the healing of the Hara Line from the energetic perspective in this chapter. Before I can do this, though, I need to describe the function of the Hara Line from the energetic perspective.

Any higher frequency energy or sentience that moves into a lower frequency is adversely affected by that frequency if is not protected in some way that allows its normal frequency of domicile to be maintained.

The Hara Line is a small energetic tube that is frequency neutral. This means that it is not affected by the frequencies that are within, or passing through, allowing it to be in many frequencies at once; it is therefore pan frequential. That which is inside this tube is therefore protected and its frequency of domicile is unaffected by the frequencies outside of the tube.

The Hara Line is small and can be considered in size terms like that of a hypodermic needle.

It is created by the TES to allow a smaller aspect of itself to be projected to any frequency that it desires without being separated from the main body of TES sentience and energy. It is mostly used in the lowest frequencies of the multiverse, for this is where it is at its most useful. This is because it allows a higher frequency to exist in a lower frequency environment without being affected adversely by that lower frequency. Although this allows the smaller aspect of TES sentience and energy, the Soul, to be maintained frequentially and therefore the connectivity with the main body of TES sentience and energy is maintained, the reduction in so-called "sentient weight" within the Hara Line reduces the communicative bandwidth down to almost nothing (while still being something!). This loss of communicative bandwidth is almost coincidental with the loss of frequency when not protected by the Hara Line or other means of low frequency protection when in a low frequency environment, and so, one can be excused for considering it as the same thing.

As stated before, the Hara Line is the connection between the TES and the individualized sentience and energy of the TES used to experience a low frequency environment via incarnation. This means that the Aspect or Soul is still joined to the TES while being protected by the Hara Line and incarnate, or associated with the incarnate vehicle, human or otherwise.

The individualized aspect of sentience and energy has its sentient weight (try to think of this in terms of air pressure within a known vessel) progressively reduced by the Hara Line as it moves down the high frequencies of the TES in its location of domicile, to the tenth frequency of the multiverse, and therefore the physical universe. The tenth frequency is also the highest of the frequencies associated with the incarnate human vehicle and is the frequential entry point for the aspect as it becomes incarnate. The sentience and associated energies then move down through the step-down function of the ninth and eighth frequencies into the energy distribution system (that starts at the seventh frequency and progresses down to the first frequency) that is used to animate the incarnate human vehicle. It stops at an area just behind the solar chakra, creating a junction point called the "Core Star." This junction sees the separation of the Aspect's sentience and its associated energies for operational purposes to two locations, the Tan Tien and the Soul Seat. The "TanTien" is the energy distribution point and is located 50 mm below the navel and 75 mm into the center of the body. The "Soul Seat" is the resting place of the sentience and is located in the area behind the front aspect of the heart chakra, close to the thymus. The total energy accumulation system (chakras) and distribution system including its junctions (mini and minor chakras) is therefore connected to the Aspect's sentience and energies via the Core Star, Tan Tien, and Soul Seat.

An energetically damaged Hara Line can cause serious health implications and even the demise of the incarnate human vehicle. This also includes the plethora of other incarnate vehicles we use in the lower frequencies of the physical universe. As a result, it is extremely important that Hara Line damage is both diagnosed and healed in an urgent and efficient way.

Damage to the Hara Line can be:

- Hara Line breach (break in tube wall)
- Hara Line inflammation
- Hara Line severance
- Hara Line disconnections (misalignment):
  - From the Soul Seat
  - From the Core Star
  - From the Tan Tien
  - From the major chakras, which ultimately includes the energetic disconnection to the minor chakras and mini chakras

## Illustration of Hara Line Damage

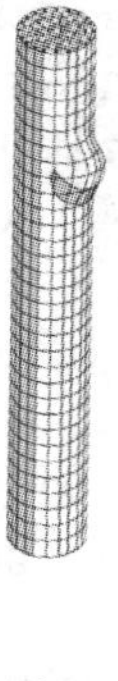

A Hara Line Bulge

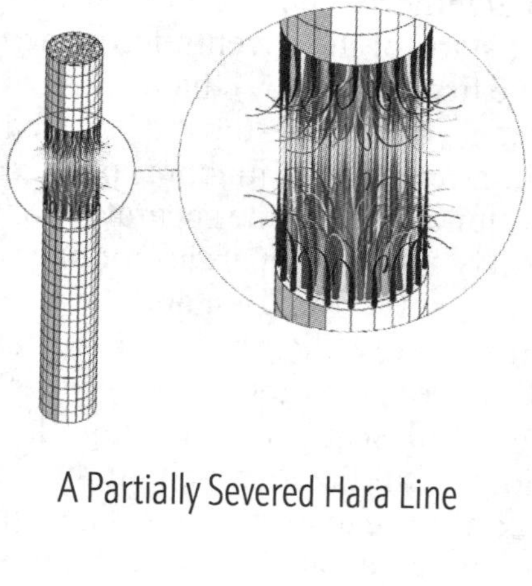

A Partially Severed Hara Line

## Healing Methods—Become Frequency Neutral

In order to heal a Hara Line breach/break in the tube wall, or indeed, any other issue with the normal functionality of the Hara Line the healer needs to assume a frequency neutral condition. If you remember, the Hara Line is a pan-frequential construct and as such is not predominantly represented on any of the frequencies associated with the incarnate human vehicle. Actually, as a construct, it originates from the frequency associated with the TES of the Aspect that occupies the incarnate human vehicle of the client. It is also likely to be a different frequency to your own Hara Lines origin. Although the Hara Line will ultimately be a much higher frequency to those of the incarnate human form, a frequency neutral condition associated with those of the incarnate human form allows the healer to heal, manipulate, or repair that part of the Hara Line that passes through them.

This being said, the healer can use the same method of attaining a neutral frequency for all clients that require their Hara Line to be healed, which is not the same as positioning yourself on all frequencies of the incarnate human vehicle concurrently as suggested could be achieved in some of the healing modalities in previous chapters, although the start of the explanation of how it is achieved is similar. This frequency neutral condition will only be functional across those frequencies that the Hara Line integrates with in reference to the incarnate human vehicle. Indeed, for healing the human Hara Line this is all we need to operate within.

To achieve a frequency neutral condition the healer must first open all of their chakras concurrently; that being, all at the same time, all in one go. This is different from opening the chakras one by one, moving up the frequencies one by one in the process. The chakras are opened by extending and spinning them clockwise all together.

Opening all of the chakras concurrently is best achieved by visualizing them extending and spinning clockwise together, all in one go, either from within the body as an extension of the healer's energies or as a diagram on a page in a book or a poster on the wall of the healing practice. If you have trouble visualizing, then use the following mentally spoken words *"I extend and spin clockwise all of my chakras in one go"* or alternatively, *"I open all of my chakras in one go."*

These visual or spoken commends will place the healer in all frequencies concurrently (pan frequentially) rather than on the frequency achieved by opening the chakras one at a time which results in predomination. For example, if the healer opens the root chakra, they are predominantly on the first frequency level. If the healer subsequently opens their sacral chakra, they are predominantly on the second frequency. If the healer then opens the solar chakra, then the heart chakra and finishes by opening the throat chakra, they will be predominantly on the fifth frequency level.

Because the Hara Line enters into the energies that construct the incarnate human vehicle at the tenth frequency the healer now needs to incorporate the eighth, ninth, and tenth frequencies into their current pan-frequential condition before creating the frequency neutral condition. To achieve this the healer needs to visualize themselves or use their mentally spoken word in order to achieve the same thing, that they are not only on the first seven frequency levels but also being on the next three frequency levels as well. One way of achieving this is to use the floors of a high-rise building to represent the frequency levels and that the healer is as tall as the number of floors (frequencies) that they are currently pan frequentially assigned to. If the healer assigns each frequency level to a floor of a high-rise building, the first frequency to the first floor, the fourth frequency to the fourth floor and so on, and that they are on all seven floors concurrently, then the healer can add in the eighth, ninth, and tenth floors into the number of floors, or frequencies that they are one with by increasing their height in relation to the number of floors in the building. Visually this illustrates that the healer is now present on ten frequency levels. However, the healer is still on all of the ten frequencies that create the incarnate human vehicle concurrently, in a pan-frequential condition rather than a frequency neutral condition.

The healer now needs to create the frequency neutral condition. This frequency neutral condition will only be relative to the ten frequencies of the incarnate human vehicle (and those of the first ten frequencies of the physical universe and, of course, the multiverse) because we have only worked with the first ten frequencies. To achieve the frequency neutral condition the healer needs to incorporate all of the ten frequencies into one composite frequency that is acceptable to all ten frequencies that the Hara Line passes through. To do this requires the healer to visualize, or use their mentally spoken word, that the image of their body is segmented in relation to the floors of the building whose floors represented the ten frequencies, that being the body has ten parts to it, like ten floors.

## Conceptual Illustration of Becoming a Neutral Frequency

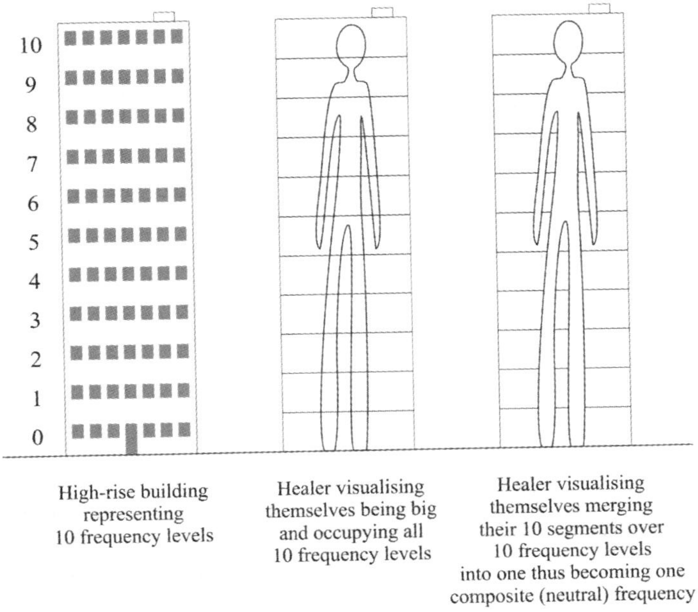

Visualize or command using your mentally spoken word that all these ten segments merge together into one. One can think of this as similar to the process of merging ten cells in a spreadsheet into one larger cell. The larger and single cell of the spreadsheet is constructed from all of the smaller cells together and so is one and all cells concurrently or is neutral to the specifics of one particular cell or frequency because it has part of it that is a particular cell to a specific cell and all other cells.

After following this process, the healer is now one composite (neutral) frequency and as such is within and without the constraints of the individual frequencies. In this neutral condition, the healer will now be able to perceive the Hara Line as an individual energy construct within the ten frequencies of the incarnate human form and will be able to affect healing, manipulation, or repairs to it directly.

To move out of the neutral frequency condition, simply reverse the process used to create the condition.

## Hara Line Inflammation

Hara Line inflammation is caused by the sentience of the incarnate aspect wanting to communicate with the TES or entities or beings within in a higher level of communicative bandwidth than is available. This in turn is created by the ego of the incarnate aspect being impatient with its spiritual development.

The inflammation is similar in representation to a bulge in a vein, tire, or inner tube, creating an area of weakness in the Hara Line and an area where the normal flow of data from the TES to the aspect and reverse is affected. This affect creates an abnormal increase in the flow of the data, followed by a decrease. In effect the Aspect feels that it has moments of increased consciousness, which leads to nothing and later creates frustration.

In order to repair such inflammation, the healer, in the neutral frequential position, can visualize the area of inflammation on the Hara Line in the same way as one of the energetic templates, like a tube that looks like a matrix that is tube shaped with the inflammation showing as a bulge on one part of the tube.

Visualize the matrix of the Hara Line and the bulge as a series of horizontal and vertical lines. Now visualize that the lines that make up the tube that is the Hara and its inflammation or bulge can be adjusted in tension. Use your intention to increase the tension on those vertical lines, those that follow the length of the Hara Line. Tighten them from the lines that are least taught, from both sides of the bulge working your way into the middle of the bulge from both sides. First one side and then the other until the tension is equal all around them. See them getting shorter around the area of the bulge with the bulge becoming smaller the more you increase the tension. Notice how the uniform shape of the Hara Line starts to return. See how the horizontal lines become slack as the vertical lines become taught, pulling the bulge in. Also notice how the slackness of the horizontal line decreases the farther away from the location of the bulge they are.

Now use your intention to tighten the tension of the horizontal lines. Work in the same way as you did with the vertical lines, working on the top and then the bottom moving in toward the center. When you reach the center lines notice how the overall shape and tension appears to be uniform, that the tube of the Hara Line is now the same shape, irrespective of where you look. With this shape now returned to normal, the normal flow of communicative spiritual data from the Aspect to the TES and vice versa is achieved and the incarnate aspect experiences no further ebbs and flows of data. Also, reduced or negated are moments of self-awareness or higher function followed by drops in these moments of higher function or self-awareness and the subsequent confusion, frustration, and depression.

## Hara Line Severance

Hara line severance is a condition when the Aspect

no longer desires to be incarnate. It is when the Hara Line no longer has a connection to either the sentience in the Soul Seat, the Tan Tien, or the Core Star. The physical representation is a disability (gained either through accident or disease) where the incarnate aspect is in a body that is paraplegic, quadriplegic, fully paralyzed (locked-in syndrome), or in a coma.

Coma is usually produced when the Soul Seat is disconnected from the Core Star but is still connected to the TES.

Full paralysis is produced in the same way but that there is incarnate consciousness.

Paraplegic and quadriplegic conditions are created when the aspect of the Hara that connects the Tan Tien to the energy distribution system and the energetic templates is partially or significantly, but not totally, severed.

Hara Kiri (traditional Japanese suicide) is another way that the Tan Tien can be fully severed from the Hara Line, effecting all energetic connectivity to the templates because the intention is to end the incarnation.

When the Hara Line is severed in one of these ways, it is difficult if not almost impossible to both reconnect the functions of the ability of the sentience within the Soul Seat to be connected to the Tan Tien to allow the connections between the Tan Tien and the energy distribution system and energetic templates to function in the way that supports animation of the incarnate human vehicle.

If the incarnate aspect is disabled as part of its life plan then the Hara Line cannot be reconnected, unless the life plan includes regaining use of the disabled limbs. In this instance, the Hara Line can be reconnected creating an opportunity for the incarnate aspect to regain the use of the limbs over time providing the incarnate aspect actually wishes to work on regaining control of the animation of the limbs.

If the incarnate aspect is fully paralyzed (not quadriplegic) then the above also applies.

If the incarnate aspect is in a coma then the aspect may not even be associated with the incarnate human vehicle it was born into. In this case the Hara Line will be totally severed and there will be no Tan Tien, Core Star, or Soul Seat. The energetic templates will be present but not active, they will appear to be dark. The human vehicle will be maintained by medical technology but not useable. It will be like a clay model. In this instance, healing is not possible.

In the event that it is part of the life plan to reintegrate with the incarnate human vehicle, or that another aspect is planning to "walk in" to the empty body, the Hara Line will be visible with the severed halves being close to each other. It will be connected but not connected, so to speak. With this is a possibility that the energy templates appear active but inert.

If the Hara Line is therefore partially severed (or connected) the healer can accelerate the return to fullness or wholeness by first placing themselves into the neutral frequency condition. Next use your visualization to see the Hara Line and the area of partial separation/connection. See it as an electric wire with a hole in the middle, with lots of strands, and that the area of severance is like the two halves of the Hara Line have been stretched and then pulled apart so that parts of the Hara Line have what appears to be stretched wires that are broken but that are thinner where the stretching has taken place by the break. Notice that the hole in the middle of the Hara is full of energy, that it bridges the gap between the severed areas; it looks like a pipe with water flowing from one part of the pipe to the other. The pipe has an internal and external diameter. The color of the energy may appear to be white, gold, and silver iridescence with flecks of energy of the same colors within the main body of the energy flow. Although the colors are simply a representation of the intensity and frequencies of the energies, they represent the combined sentience and energy that is the projected Aspect (Soul) from the True Energetic Self (TES) into the incarnate human vehicle. The severed "wires" of the outside of the tube of wires represent the connectivity of the Hara with the Tan Tien and Soul Seat via the Core Star.

Note that the area of the Hara that is also a little stretched but not to the point where it has resulted in separation has "wires" that are thinner but not severed. One can also consider that these wires are similar to a large number of nerves, or tendrils, with some of the nerves or tendrils still being connected to each other.

Now use your intuition to look at each of the severed wires (nerves/tendrils) and look at which one on one side of the break is the same as one of the severed wires (nerves/tendrils) on the other side of the break. At first glance they may look the same or similar but look closely and you will see that they are specific to each other, just like the colors of the insulation on multicore wire, such as data or telephone wire. There will be any number of these wires/nerves/tendrils that are both connected or severed. Those that are not severed but are stretched can be left alone.

Now work on those that are severed. Visualize those wires/nerves/tendrils that are severed moving together one at a time one "color or type" at a time. Use your intention to merge those wires/nerves/tendrils of the outer diameter of the Hara Line joining together again. Think of them as being one and not two halves. You can consider them welding together if you like.

As you merge each one you will notice that the inside and outside diameters of the Hara Line—the hose of the pipe or outer insulation of the multicore wire in this example—get closer and closer together, merging and welding, as more of the wires/nerves/tendrils of the structure of the Hara Line are merged together.

Once all of the wires/nerves/tendrils of the structure of the Hara are merged together (healed) the rest of the outer part (the outer insulation or hose in the examples) finally merges together as one. Once this has been achieved the normal connectivity with the Core Star, Tan Tien, and Soul Seat will be resumed.

Once the energetics of the Hara Line are

reestablished the normal abilities of the aspect to animate the incarnate human vehicle are available. Available, that is, if it is in the life plan to be available. If full animation is not in the life plan, then either no animation or a small improvement may be witnessed. Psycho-spiritually the patient may experience more resolve, personal direction, and motivation to "get on with life." This in itself is the most important aspect of healing that you can offer as a healer for increased motivation/resolve and end desire/intention can be healing in its own right.

## Hara Line Disconnections (misalignment)

Hara Line disconnections can also be described as misalignment or disharmony (not being in tune). They are not total or partial severance of the Hara Line from any of the major connections, such as the Core Star, Soul Seat, Tan Tien, and the chakras as described in the previous section above.

Misalignment is also not a physical misalignment of the tube that is the Hara Line with the major connections; it is more psycho-spiritual because it includes the intention behind the connections and the harmony or alignment of the frequencies associated with those connections. In essence, the frequencies are matched to each other and are not out of "phase" so to speak. If they are even slightly out of alignment or harmony, then the functions of the major connections will not work correctly, including the intentions behind them. Although misalignment is not a physical image of two connections not being quite connected per se, the healer may well see this type of image in their spiritual vision or mind's eye. They may be given this as a representation of what is happening with the patient, which of course draws the attention of the healer to the need to heal Hara Line misalignment in the area where this imagery is located.

All disconnections can be healed by psycho-spiritual healing; that being, the intention can be changed by changing the desire behind the intention, which creates correct thought and subsequently correct actions. The following psycho-spiritual intentions are relative to the major Hara Line connections:

- From the Soul Seat is the intention to be in the physical
- From the Core Star is the intention to be connected to the physical
- From the Tan Tien is the intention to move in or interact with the physical
- From the major chakras is the intention to maintain the energies of the incarnate human vehicle.
- From the minor chakras is the intention to distribute the energies of the incarnate human vehicle.
- From mini chakras is the intention to animate the incarnate human vehicle.

To change these intentions is to change the alignment and create harmonious frequential connectivity and communication between all areas of the energy templates and the gross physical aspect of the incarnate human vehicle.

Changing the intention of the patient is a function of "psycho-spiritual" healing or reprogramming. Although this is described in more detail in a chapter of its own, and as a result uses a more comprehensive method, the basis of this healing modality can be used to heal Hara Line disconnections or misalignments.

In order to affect an intentional change in the psycho-spiritual programming of the patient and correct a Hara Line disconnection or misalignment the healer must create a condition between themselves and the patient where the healer can visualize the psycho-spiritual programming of the patient in a way that they find easy to work with. In my personal experience I have changed from a number of visualization methods over the years, and the simplest version that I have used is one where I see myself at the desk of a series of switches. This desk of switches being the basic psycho-spiritual programming associated with the patient.

First, though, place yourself in the frequency neutral position described in the last section and when you have achieved this you can use your visualization (or your mentally spoken words) to create a room. In order to enter into the patient's psycho-spiritual programming see yourself within this room.

The room is the patient's psycho-spiritual programming; in totality, every aspect of the patient's psycho-spiritual programming can be accessed in this room. Within this room you visualize a desk of psycho-spiritual switches that are the basic programming of the patient's intention relative to the alignment of the Hara Line with its major connections. The desk of switches has a simple ON/OFF function. Each of the switches in this desk are associated with a different intention, which can therefore be turned on or off, effectively changing the psycho-spiritual direction of the incarnate aspect and therefore the way they operate within their incarnation in terms of with themselves and those that they interact with within their environment.

Now create another visualization. See above the desk of switches a large display screen. In this display screen, place an image of the patient's energy system relative to the Hara Line. The connections of the Hara Line exist from the TES to the Core Star, the Tan Tien, and the Soul Seat. Also visualize the energy lines from the Tan Tien to the major, minor, and mini chakras as separate from, but ultimately connected to, the Hara via the Tan Tien and therefore affected by the Hara Line. The connection between the major chakras is via a major energy conduit. The connection between the major energy conduit and the minor chakras is via minor energy lines. The connections between the minor energy lines and the mini chakras is via mini energy lines.

Now visualize the desk of switches in more detail. There will be six switches.

There will be:

1. One ON/OFF switch for the connection from the Hara Line to Core Star. Label this switch with the words "intention to be connected to the physical."
2. One ON/OFF switch for the connection from the Core Star to the Soul Seat. Label this switch with the words "intention to be in the physical."
3. One ON/OFF switch for the connection from the Core Star to the Tan Tien. Label this switch with the words "intention to move in, or interact with, the physical."
4. One ON/OFF switch for the connection from the Tan Tien to the major energy conduit that connects the major chakras together and to the Tan Tien. Label this switch with the words "intention to maintain the energies of the incarnate human vehicle."
5. One ON/OFF switch for the connection from the major chakras through the major energy conduit that connects the major chakras together to the minor energy lines that connect the minor chakras to the major energy conduit. Label this switch with the words "intention to distribute the energies of the incarnate human vehicle."
6. One ON/OFF switch for the connection from the minor chakras through the minor energy lines that connects the minor chakras together to the mini energy lines that connect the mini chakras to the minor energy lines. Label this switch with the words "intention to animate

the incarnate human vehicle."

The healer should now look closely at the image of the energy systems of the patient that they have projected onto the display. If any of these energetic connections look misaligned in any way then that reflects a psycho-spiritual issue with the patient. This should be observable in the way they think, behave, and act.

Misalignment can appear like the Hara Line is trying to avoid being directly connected to the location that it is supposed to be connected to, such as the Tan Tien or Soul Seat. It may appear distorted or bent in some cases. A distortion gives the appearance of being hazy and results in a lack of clear thinking, behaving, and acting. A bend in the Hara Line results in aversion to thinking, behaving, and acting.

Let us consider that the patient we are looking at displays all of the conditions identified above. Although it is highly unlikely that a patient will actually present all of these psycho-spiritual "symptoms," it is a remote possibility. Based upon this, it is possible that, in an extreme case, you may well be presented with a patient that is in very poor physical and mental health. In this instance, all of their switches will be in the "OFF" position.

While in the room that represents the patient's psycho-spiritual programming visualize yourself seeing the desk of switches and the image on the display of the patient in front of you. Further visualize yourself moving the switch that represents the connection from the Core Star to the Soul Seat from off to on. This is the patient's intention to be incarnate. Once you have done this you will need to assign this "change in state" to all of the seven templates that are used to create the incarnate human vehicle. This is a necessary requirement for all psycho-spiritual programming because the reprogramming needs to affect all aspects of the incarnate human vehicle, on all the main frequencies associated with it. To achieve this, visualize another group of eight switches. Seven of the switches are relative to the seven frequencies associated with the seven energetic templates. The eighth is an "overall" save function. Each of the seven switches will also have two states, ON or OFF. The eighth associated with the overall save function has two different states, "NOT SAVED" and "SAVED."

Using your intention change the state of the seven switches from off to on. Change the state individually starting from the switch marked 1 (the etheric body) moving through the switch marked 2 (the emotional layer), 3 (mental body), 4 (astral level), 5 (etheric template), 6 (celestial body), to 7 (ketheric template). Once you have changed the state of all seven energetic templates you can now create the final assignation by changing the state of the eighth switch to "saved."

You have now changed the intention of the patient to be in the physical. You will also note that the connection between the Hara Line and the Soul Seat is now direct. Any appearance of misalignment will have been removed. The Hara Line and its connection to the Core Star will be straight and clearly in focus, it will not be diffuse.

You can now use this process to change the intention of the patient to remain connected to the physical by reestablishing the connection between the Hara Line and the Core Star.

Or …

change the intention of the patient to interact or move in the physical by reestablishing the connection between the Core Star and the Tan Tien.

Or …

change the intention of the patient to maintain the energies of the incarnate human vehicle by reestablishing the connection between the Tan Tien and the major chakras.

Or …

change the intention of the patient to distribute the energies of the incarnate human vehicle by reestablishing the connection between the major chakras and the minor chakras.

Or ...

change the intention of the patient to animate the incarnate human vehicle by reestablishing the connection between the minor chakras and the mini chakras.

In each of these cases the connections from the higher function to the lower function (for example, the Tan Tien to the major chakras) will be straight or direct and clearly in focus.

At the end of this process you should change your state from being in the neutral frequential condition to that which you normally are when not performing the service of being a healer.

# Removing Karmic Links

Karmic links have two classifications. Those that are between two incarnate aspects or Souls and those that are between the incarnate aspect and itself. Karmic links that are between the incarnate aspect and itself are not to be confused with links that are between the incarnate aspect in this current incarnation and those of a previous incarnation. These are defined as removing past life links and have previously been discussed.

Karmic links can be dissolved or removed by the incarnate aspects or with the help of an experienced healer.

To elaborate further in the description of these two classifications …

## Karmic Links between Two Separate or Different Aspects

Karmic links between two separate or different aspects can be created and dissolved in the current incarnation. Also, karmic links between two separate or different aspects can be carried over from previous incarnations if not resolved and can therefore be dissolved in this incarnation.

This karmic link is between the incarnate aspects of the True Energetic Self (TES) and not between the TES of the incarnate aspects. This is correct even though the TES themselves are linked to the smaller individualized sentience and energy they have separated out from themselves to create the incarnate aspect (of themselves) to experience, learn, and evolve by temporarily associating this small part of themselves with the lowest frequencies of the multiverse, within the physical universe, through the process of incarnation.

Karmic links can be created in any of the frequencies associated with the physical universe and in any of the incarnate vehicles that are available within it. Karma is therefore not limited to those aspects that use the human incarnate vehicle to experience, learn, and evolve. Karma is, however, limited to the physical universe and its frequencies.

## Karmic Links between the Aspect and Itself

Karmic links between the incarnate aspect and itself can be further subdivided into two classifications: low frequency thoughts, behaviors, and actions carried over from a previous incarnation that have not been recognized and changed; and low frequency thoughts, behaviors, and actions that we have been attracted to in the current incarnation and that have not been recognized and changed (see cyclic and downward spiraling karma in my book *Avoiding Karma*).

In both of these two karmic situations the links can be dissolved in this current incarnation without the need to refer to a past life. This is because we are not dealing with past life trauma but with the way in which the patient relates to their environment, the temptations and potential addictions within that environment, and those other incarnate aspects that they interact with within their environment/s.

**Karmic links between the Aspect and Itself from a previous incarnation are usually via the heart chakra but can include all chakras.**

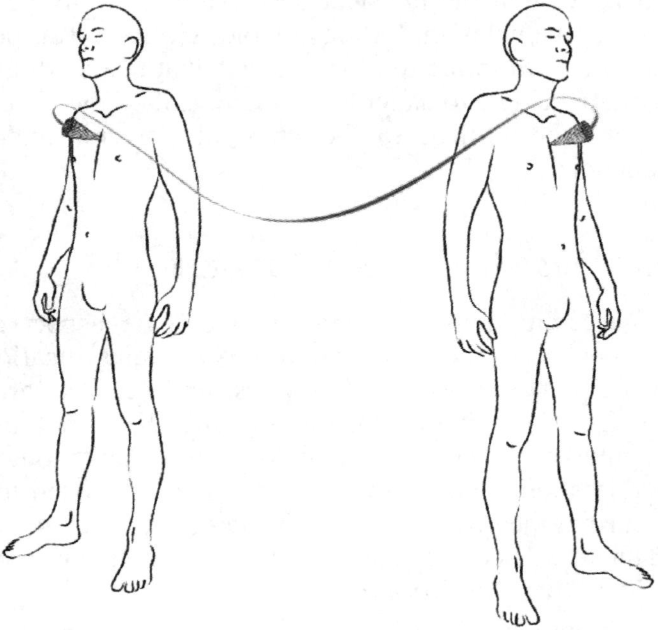

## Removing Karmic Links between Two Seperate or Different Aspects

There are two main ways in which the healer can affect the dissolution of a karmic link between two separate or different incarnate aspects. Both ways require the healer and the patient to work together in tandem to be fully effective. It must be noted first, though, that the healer must have diagnosed a karmic link between the patient and another, usually by scanning them, before continuing to work in this way. As a useful double check, the healer should conduct an independent scan of the patient looking for such links even if the patient says they feel they have one.

The first one requires the healer to be a facilitator,

the patient dissolving the link themselves by giving or requesting forgiveness. In the second way, the healer positions themselves as an energetic observer and visualizes the link as an energetic thread between the patient and the incarnate aspect that the patient is karmically attached or linked to and then removes it.

## Seeking and Giving Forgiveness

In facilitating the giving of forgiveness, the healer asks the patient to close their eyes and feel the link or connection between them and the other, sometimes unknown incarnate aspect. In feeling this link the patient may start to feel emotions surrounding the link or connection. In the event that the patient is the cause of the link then the healer needs to lead the patient into a process of seeking forgiveness from the incarnate aspect that they are linked to. They need to say a meaningful sentence that they can believe in and know is a true request for forgiveness and not just repeat the words that the healer gives them to repeat. In order to arbitrate this, the healer should ideally ask the patient to create the meaningful sentence themselves. This gives it more credibility and psycho-spiritual weight, so to speak. In speaking this meaningful sentence, the patient needs to see it, feel it, know it, be it—with their whole being.

Once this process is done, the patient may experience a change in their demeanor either straight away or over a short to medium period. The faster the request for forgiveness is received by the receiver of any wrongdoing by the patient, the faster the request for forgiveness will be accepted and the "weight" of the karmic link removed from the patient.

Most individuals (patients) will not recognize the need to ask for forgiveness as a function of their healing, specifically if it has been carried over from a previous incarnation and may therefore offer resistance. In this instance, it is the job of the healer to advise the patient that in order to be healed they need to accept responsibility for that which they have done to others in this or previous incarnations.

The reciprocal of the above is the need to give forgiveness to another incarnate aspect who has wronged us in some way. Most patients will find this difficult, especially if they have been abused in some way in this incarnation. They may have even more trouble relating to the need to give forgiveness to another incarnate aspect who wronged them in some way in a previous incarnation, simply because they will have no reference point to work from. In this case it is the role of the healer, as the result of the normal process of scanning the patient to advise them of the link and the need to dissolve it. In this instance, the healer needs to exercise diplomacy in how they broadcast this need.

In the case of giving forgiveness to another incarnate aspect that had wronged them in a previous incarnation, the healer can use the same process as above but changing the meaning behind the words from seeking forgiveness to giving forgiveness. Again, this needs to be performed in a positive and meaningful way, where the patient thinks, feels, knows, and is in total forgiveness.

Note that any doubt or feeling of retribution no matter how small is enough to negate or significantly reduce the effectiveness of the forgiveness and the depth of dissolution of the link.

In the case of giving forgiveness to an individual who has wronged or abused the patient in some way in the current incarnation, the healer needs to first scan the patient in order to see or visualize the links and ask the patient to describe the conditions and circumstances surrounding the wrongdoing or abuse. Care should be taken to ensure that the patient is not overtly emotionally stressed as some descriptions may be graphic, disturbing, or frightening to the patient, especially if they relive the experience as a result of describing it. If this is the case, the healer should be sympathetic and may need to break down the forgiveness process into achievable parts.

So long as the patient is stable, the healer can guide

the patient through the process of giving forgiveness. Ask the patient to close their eyes and visualize the face or faces of the individual/s whom they are going to forgive. Then explain to them that the incarnate aspect who wronged or abused them is a Soul, just the same as them, struggling to experience, learn, and evolve just the same as them. You may also explain that both the patient and the wrongdoer may have worked together to create this experience. However, if you feel that this is a step too far, it's best to leave this part of the process out.

Create a meaningful sentence for the patient to use in order to administer forgiveness. First, you say it out loud and then ask the patient to repeat it. The healer needs to reiterate the importance of the forgiveness being given in a positive and meaningful way, where the patient thinks, feels, knows, and is in total unconditional forgiveness. As with giving forgiveness to an aspect from a past life, forgiveness needs to be given without any doubt or hidden feelings of spite or retribution, otherwise it will be limited in its effectiveness and may not be enough to dissolve the link between the patient and the wrongdoer/s. If multiple wrongdoers are involved, then all faces and names must be visualized to negate any group-based karma between the patient and the wrongdoers.

It must be noted by the healer that even if one of the wrongdoers is left out from the patient's list of those he/she must forgive then the group karma will not be dissolved. Based upon this, creating a forgiveness list of the names and faces must be inclusive rather than exclusive when being compiled.

This is a very powerful way to dissolve karmic links between two incarnate aspects, indeed it is the most effective if performed with full meaning and full unreserved and unconditional forgiveness.

## Forgiving Oneself

Forgiving oneself can be a particularly difficult task to do specifically when one does not know what one needs to forgive oneself for. A specific example of lack of recognition of the need to forgive oneself is when we have done something wrong or made a mistake and no one else is or has been affected. For example, we may chastise ourselves for scratching the paintwork on our car, our thought processes going in circles as to why we scratched the paintwork and how we should have avoided the event that created it. The more we think about it, the more we get frustrated with ourselves, with the frustration limiting our ability to see a bigger picture, that bigger picture being the ability to experience, learn, and evolve from a certain action, and if necessary, forgive ourselves for any errors, irrespective of how big or small they are.

In order to understand what the patient needs to forgive themselves or indeed others for, the healer must ask the patient questions about their activities in and around the time that they started to become ill or unwell, to determine which thought, behavior, and action needs to be forgiven.

The thought, behavior, and action may be considered to be insignificant to both the healer and the patient, but this is not an indication of the effect on the gross physical aspect of the incarnate human vehicle. As such, every possibility no matter how small must be considered as something that needs to be forgiven.

Once you have established ALL of the possibilities that the patient needs to forgive themselves for, you can commence with the healing. As with forgiving another, the healing process requires active participation by the patient to ensure that the healing created by self-forgiveness is successful.

Ask the patient to close their eyes and mentally focus on the memory of the thought, behavior, and action of the item of personal activity that is the cause of the illness. In the event that there are many individual thoughts, behaviors, and actions that contribute to either one total illness or a number of smaller illnesses, then the thought, behavior, and action that has the biggest impact must be worked with first. The others must be worked on in order of impact or priority. For the benefit of this book, though, we will assume that there is only one overall thought, behavior, and action that needs to be worked on.

With the patient's eyes closed, ask them to visualize the thought, behavior, and action that is the root cause of the physical illness or dysfunction. Also, visualize it yourself. Ask the patient to replay the thought, behavior, and action as a scenario, ask them to repeat what they are seeing verbally.

When the patient gets to the part in the scenario that they feel could be better you can start to assist them by advising them that how they thought, behaved, and acted was appropriate. That it was based upon a number of factors that were available at the time of the thoughts, behaviors, and actions. That the reaction to the need to respond to a circumstance, individual or a circumstance and subsequential interaction with an individual in a certain environment was the best that they could have achieved, at that time, without the power of hindsight. That what they did was perfect.

Ask the patient to repeat out loud that this was the very best that they could have done, that comparing their current version to their past version cannot be used to confirm the level of success. Ask them to repeat a series of powerful words to make them feel, be, and know that this is true and that this was the very best outcome possible at that time. Make the patient repeat the words out loud while visualizing the situation. Tell them to see forgiveness, be forgiveness, and know forgiveness.

As they visualize and verbalize the thought, behavior, and action that created the physical illness or dysfunction, visualize the link between the current version of themselves and the previous version. Then visualize yourself removing this link like removing an electric cable by disconnecting the plugs between the patient and their former selves. Now visualize your recycling bin and placing the link, this electric cable, into the bin. This effectively severs the link, but it doesn't stop it from being reconnected. To stop any reconnections from occurring, visualize the connections like an electric socket on a wall and that both the current and previous versions of the patient have a socket on their body. Remove each socket in turn from the current and previous version of the patient in the same way as you would remove a socket from a wall in your house. This should be done by removing the socket's retaining screws, then disconnecting wires that are in the wall from the socket, insulating the wires with insulating tape, and then sealing the wall by plastering the aperture where the socket was. This effectively stops any further reconnections with the patient and the previous version of the patient and reestablishing the dissatisfaction with the product of the thoughts, behaviors, and actions. With this visualization process complete and the patient removing the comparison with the current and previous versions of themselves the illness or dysfunction will start to dissolve, and the patient will return to health. It is usual to see an improvement straight after the healing process has been completed but deeper associations with the previous self can take a couple of weeks to dissolve.

Once completed you can ask the patient to open their eyes slowly, come back into the room, and take a drink of water. The healing is finished.

## Removing the Karmic Links from a Wrongdoer

Actually, the detail behind the process, described above, of forgiving oneself by removing karmic links between the patient and himself/herself can be used with great success when forgiving others. However, if a number of individuals are involved then they will need to be forgiven one by one and with the individual that causes the biggest illness or physical dysfunction being given priority with the remaining individuals being forgiven in a descending order of priority.

Although mostly a repeat of the pervious description, the text below can be of assistance in removing a karmic link with another person or a wrongdoer.

With the patient's eyes closed, ask them to visualize

the thought, behavior, and action that is the root cause of the karmic link with another, created by the other or by the patient. Also, visualize it yourself. Ask the patient to replay the behaviors and actions of the wrongdoer or themselves as a scenario, and ask the patient to repeat what they are seeing verbally.

When the patient gets to the part in the scenario that they feel is the issue that created the karmic link you can start to assist them by advising them that how they both thought, behaved, and acted was appropriate. That it was based upon a number of factors that were available at the time. That the reaction to the need to respond to a circumstance and subsequential interaction with an individual in a certain environment was consequential and needed no aggressive interaction. Ask the patient to repeat out loud that this was not a big issue. Ask them to repeat a series of powerful words to make them feel, be, and know that this is true. Make the patient repeat the words out loud while visualizing the situation. Tell them to see forgiveness, be forgiveness, and know forgiveness and that the link needs to be removed by one of them and that they, the patient, would like to remove it, benefiting both of them.

As they visualize and verbalize the circumstance that created the karmic link, visualize the link between the current version of themselves and the other incarnate aspect. Then visualize yourself removing this link like removing an electric cable by disconnecting the plugs between the patient and the other incarnate aspect. Now visualize your recycling bin and placing the link, this electric cable, into the bin. This effectively severs the link, but it doesn't stop it from being reconnected. To stop any reconnections from occurring, visualize the connections like an electric socket on a wall and that both the current and previous versions of the other incarnate aspect (patient) have a socket on their body. Remove each socket in turn from the current and the other incarnate aspect in the same way as you would remove a socket from a wall in your house. This should be done by removing the socket's retaining screws, then disconnecting wires that are in the wall from the socket, insulating the wires with insulating tape, and then sealing the wall by plastering the aperture where the socket was. This effectively stops any further reconnections with the patient and the other incarnate aspect and the possibility of reestablishing the karmic link. With this visualization process complete and you removing the karmic link, the patient will return to health. It is usual to see an improvement straight after the healing process has been completed but deeper associations with the other incarnate aspect can take a couple of weeks to dissolve.

# Removing Foreign Objects

The removal of a foreign object from either the energetic templates or human energy field (aura) of the incarnate human vehicle is a similar process, if not the same, as removing a foreign object from a chakra, which was illustrated earlier in this book.

However, to remove a foreign object from either one or all of the energetic templates or layers of the human energy field, the healer must first establish that there is an issue that can be related to a foreign object. This is achieved by scanning the patient's body, energy system, and aura. Second, the detailed analysis is performed one frequency at a time, by the healer opening their chakras one chakra at a time, so that each of the energy templates and auric layers associated with the chakra being opened can be observed and analyzed. This is to ensure that only the auric layer/s or energy template/s that needs/need to be worked on is/are in fact worked on, that the energetic representation of the foreign object is recognized, and the scope of the work needed to remove it is established.

Once all of the above has been established, the healer can commence the task of removing the foreign object from the energy template/s and/or auric layer/s identified. It does have to be noted, though, that in many cases the foreign object rarely penetrates just one auric layer or energy template. Additionally, it rarely penetrates any energy template without first penetrating all seven auric layers, although a foreign object can penetrate all seven layers of the auric layer without penetrating any energy template. Finally, it must also be noted that in all of the cases that I have experienced, the foreign object is normally represented on all of the frequency levels of the energy templates that it has penetrated. This means that although the object has penetrated all seven auric layers it may only have penetrated the first three energy templates, levels seven, six, and five, for example. As a result, the healer will only need to remove the foreign object on these levels; this means that the healer will need to open all chakras and work on removing the foreign object as it is represented on the seventh frequency within the seventh energy template, then close the seventh chakra and work on removing the foreign object as it is represented on the sixth frequency within the sixth energy template, then close the sixth chakra and work on removing the foreign object as it is represented on the fifth frequency within the fifth energy template. This is not necessary with the auric layers (see below).

The first energy template to work on is the seventh as this is the one that a foreign object would come in contact with first, and as a result it is the frequential opposite of working on repairing or replacing the chakras, for example. Therefore, the healer needs to open all seven chakras first and then close them down one by one as they remove the foreign object as it is represented on each frequency level from each energy template, in descending order. However, when working with the aura, although the healer needs to elevate their own frequencies to the seventh level to remove the foreign object from the seventh auric layer, they can stay on the seventh frequency to work on ALL the auric layers and not descend the frequencies to remove the foreign object from the lower frequencies of the auric layers.

There are two reasons for this.

First, the auric layers are amorphous in comparison to the energy templates because they are a byproduct of the work of the chakras and therefore have limited structure (even though they can be used as a defensive energetic shield!). Second, the energy templates are specific in their structure because they dictate the form and function of the incarnate human vehicle.

## Removing a Foreign Object from the Auric Layers

When working on removing a foreign object from the auric layers, the healer must elevate to the seventh frequency by opening all seven chakras.

Using visualization (clairvoyance), the healer should observe how the foreign object is attached or lodged within the aura and which auric layers are affected.

Once the healer has elevated himself to the seventh frequency level and has visualized the energy affecting the auric layer in the way it has presented itself to the healer as a foreign object (see the chapter on removing a foreign object from the chakras), the healer can then establish how best to remove that object.

The healer should work on removing the foreign object as if it is solid, visualizing using the hands to gently move the object out of the auric layer/s. The auric layers should be treated with care ensuring that the removal of the object doesn't create more damage in the process of removing it than has already been caused by it. If need be, the healer should twist and turn the object to avoid tearing any of the gossamer-like structure of the auric layers. Again, as with foreign objects embedded within the chakras, I have seen foreign objects that have barbs like fishhooks which can tear the auric layers, cutting them like rice paper. Do not try to break the foreign object to assist in its removal as this will allow some of the energies associated with it to disperse around the auric layers of the patient, which will need to be cleaned and cleared. It cannot be left within the energies of the patient because it will create residual issues associated with the foreign object. Once the object has been removed, it can be discarded into a recycling bin that the healer can manifest close by to them using their intention to make sure that anything that is placed within it is sent back to The Source.

The auric layers can be repaired by considering

them as a series of seven super-fine 3D grids or nets, the damaged areas being represented by tears in the 3D grids or nets. To repair this 3D grid or net, the healer should visualize reconnecting the tears with the undamaged aspects of the grid or net. One example of how to reconnect the tears is to visualize stitching or darning the damaged area to the good area in a similar way that one would darn or repair an item of clothing. The healer will observe a change in the appearance of the auric layer when the 3D grid or net is repaired. Noting that the healer needs to remain on the seventh frequency (all seven chakras open) the healer should work on the first auric layer first and then repair the other auric layers, two through seven, in an ascending order. Once completed the healer can then descend the frequencies back to the Earth level, taking a drink of water to ground himself.

## Removing a Foreign Object from the Energetic Templates

When working on removing a foreign object from the energetic templates the healer must also note that they will need to affect healing on the auric layers, as noted above, at the very end of the work on the energy templates.

The healer will need to elevate to the seventh frequency by opening all seven chakras and using visualization (clairvoyance); the healer should observe how the foreign object is attached or lodged within the energetic templates noting which are affected. If the foreign object is only lodged within one energetic template, the first to be affected is the seventh, then the healer will only need to work on removing the object from that template. If, however, the object is also interfering with (impaled within) other energetic templates, then the healer will need to ensure that they also remove the object from the remaining energetic templates affected in a descending order, six through to one if all are affected.

Once the healer has elevated himself to the correct frequency level and has visualized the energy affecting the energy template in the way it has presented itself to the healer as a foreign object in one of the ways previously described, the healer can then establish how best to remove that object.

As previously stated, the healer should work on removing the foreign object as if it is solid, visualizing using the hands to gently move the object out of the energetic template. The energy template should be treated with the same care as a consultant surgeon would treat the incarnate human vehicles physical skin, ensuring that they don't create more damage in removing the object than has already been caused by it. If need be, the healer should twist and turn the object to avoid tearing any of the small 3D energy lines or grids that represent the energy template on the level you are working on. Don't forget that these foreign objects can be complex or represent a weapon of some sort. For example, I have seen foreign objects that look like knives, swords, or spears as well as those that have barbs like fishhooks which can tear the energy lines of the energetic template. The object can be twisted and turned in order to remove it. Do not try to break the foreign object to assist in its removal as this will allow some of the energies associated with it to disperse around the energetic template and chakra of the patient on that level, which will need to be cleaned and cleared as previously stated. It cannot be left within the energies of the patient because it will create residual issues associated with the foreign object. Once the object has been removed, it can be discarded into a recycling bin that the healer can manifest close by to them using their intention to make anything that is placed within it get sent back to The Source.

Once the object has been removed, the healer needs to descend to the sixth frequency to work on the sixth energetic template by closing the seventh chakra (crown), for example.

Continue down the energetic templates affected by the foreign object in the frequentially descending order until the foreign object is removed from all energetic templates affected. Ensure that all residual energies from the foreign object are cleansed and cleared away. This can be done by the healer visualizing the damaged area being surrounded or bathed in silver light. In the gross physical, silver has antibacterial and antimicrobial properties. In the metaphysical, it can act as a sterilizing agent and actively promote healing. I use it to cleanse and sterilize the damaged areas of all aspects of the incarnate human vehicle.

Once cleansed, the energetic templates can be repaired by considering it as a 3D grid or net, the damaged areas being represented by tears in the 3D grid or net. To repair this 3D grid or net, the healer should visualize reconnecting the tears with the undamaged aspects of the grid or net. Repairs to the energetic templates should be performed from the lowest frequency template affected and then in an ascending order up to the highest or seventh. One example of how to reconnect the tears is to visualize stitching or darning the damaged area to the good area in a similar way that one would darn or repair an item of clothing. Once the lowest frequency energetic template is repaired—for example, the second energy template—the healer can elevate their own frequency to the third frequency by opening the third chakra (solar) to allow them to work on the third energetic template and continue to work in an ascending order.

The healer will observe a change in the appearance of an energetic template when the 3D grid or net is repaired. As stated before I usually see the template glow iridescently.

Once all the energetic templates have had the foreign object removed from them, and have been repaired, the healer must then work on repairing the tears in the auric layers using the methods specified above before completing the healing by descending the frequencies (closing the chakras in descending order) to the Earth level and taking a drink of water to ground themselves.

# Removing Links with Other Incarnates (Non-Karmic)

It is a common function of interacting with other incarnates, whether on the Earth or other planetary environments within the physical universe, that we create a link of some sort with them. Many of these links are created within the current incarnation and not those from previous incarnations. These links may not actually be based upon a karmic situation either. Some links are naturally acceptable or desirable while some can be considered detrimental or nonessential to the incarnate aspect and its evolutionary experience in this incarnation.

Such links may be with:

- Parents
- Partners
- Children
- Friends
- Work associates
- Pastime associates
- Permanent(within the incarnation) associations from any of the above
- Transient associations from any of the above

It would be reasonable to consider that links between incarnate aspects that are classified as being acceptable or desirable are not usually something that a patient would need to have removed or that their removal would play an active part in their healing process. It would also be reasonable to assume that a link that is classified as being detrimental would need to be removed—without question. However, this may not always be the case and the healer needs to ask the guide and helpers of the patient for the relevance of the links after establishing who they are associated with before deciding to remove them. Once the relevance of the link is established, the healer can then decide to remove them as part of the healing process or not.

To assist the healer in gaining the relevance of the link or links, the healer needs to ask the patient a series of questions to further establish the physical or psycho-spiritual effects of the links being in place.

Basic questions aligned to the links should establish if:

- It creates a physical dysfunction? (unlikely but could be due to psychological stress)
- It creates a psychological dysfunction? (most likely and will create some form or level of stress)
- The patient has problems with:
    a. Family issues? Such as:
        i. Parents?
        ii. Siblings?
        iii. In-Laws?
        iv. Their partner?
        v. Issues with their children?
    b. Extra family issues such as:
        i. Previous marriage partners?
        ii. Previous marriage children?
        iii. Previous marriage in-laws?
    c. Issues with work colleagues?
    d. Issues with friends?
    e. Depression?
    f. Emotions that result in:
        i. anxiety?

ii. tiredness?
iii. extremes in emotional responses?
iv. problems with temper or calmness?
v. problems with ownership/ responsibility?

Once the healer has worked with these questions and recognized that the issue/s the patient is facing and the direction, or directions, that they are coming from are relative to links with certain individuals, the healer can then embark upon removing these links.

Moreover, the healer now has a focal point. This being:

- The issue is based upon a link with another incarnate.
- The link affects the way in which the patient interacts with others.
- That no karma is involved.
- The link is detrimental, or not—but has a need to be removed.

Furnished with the answers to the questions above, the healer now has to connect with the patient by raising their own frequencies to that of the seventh level by opening all of their chakras one by one. This will allow them to connect with the patient on all seven levels concurrently, negating the need to work on one level and then the next level, etc.

## Removing the Links with Another

Having established that there is a link to another individual or individuals and the effects it has on the patient, the healer can work upon the task of severing that link.

As previously stated, some healers who sever

links generally only do that and miss the fact that this link can, and normally does, reestablish itself upon a later date. Based upon this, the healer needs to not only remove the link, but also the method of linking the patient to the other individual/s. The healer performs this task from the seventh frequency level by opening the chakras as previously mentioned. If there is more than one link between the patient and an individual, the healer should perform the task of removing the links using the method below one by one until they are sufficiently skilled and confident to take on the task of removing all links at the same time. If there is more than one individual involved, the healer should remove the link or links from one individual one at a time (or all together if sufficiently skilled and confident) and only then move on to removing the link or links (see above) from the next individual that the patient is linked to. An extremely experienced healer can remove all links from all individuals that the patient is linked to at the same time.

While on the seventh level, the healer needs to visualize the patient and the other individual/s that they are linked to. The healer will see a link (or links), an energy line (or lines), between some part of the incarnate human vehicle that is the patient and some part of the other individual/s that are linked to it.

The healer should also visualize the recycling bin used in previous descriptions.

As previously described, although I visualize the link between the two incarnates as being an electric cable with a plug on either end of the cable, it is clearly an energetic link. The link is connected to the energies of the incarnate vehicles used by the patient and the individual/s it is linked to. It manifests as a lump of energy on each of the seven energetic/frequential templates of the patient integrating them in an adaptive way with the link and the seven energetic/frequential templates of the individual/s they are linked to.

Using my illustration, each plug is connected to a socket on the body of each incarnate vehicle, rather like an electric socket on the wall of your house.

Visualize removing the plug (male connection) from each end of the cable (link) from the socket (female connection) on the body of the incarnate vehicle of the patient and the incarnate vehicle of the other person. Deposit the cable and plugs into your energy recycling bin. This simply severs the link between the patient and the other individual. However, as stated above it only severs the link and not the connectivity. If the connectivity between the patient and the other individual is not removed as well, the link can be reestablished recreating the issues that were previously invoked by such a link.

Continuing to use the theme of the electrical plugs, cable, and wall socket (female connection) to remove the link, the healer should now concentrate on removing the sockets on the bodies (the incarnate vehicles) of the patient and the other individual. I use the visualization of unscrewing the faceplate of the socket and then removing the wires from the faceplate before terminating the wires correctly in an electrically secure way such as using terminal blocks (a way of connecting electrical wires together —GSN) and wrapping insulation tape around them. I then visualize backfilling the remaining hole with energy so that the hole no longer exists. If one uses the visualization of filling the patras (where the socket is embedded into the wall) with plaster, as in the example that the socket was on a wall in your house, then you have created a solid block of energy that stops the possibility of reconnecting with a new link. Provided, that is, that both sockets on the patient and the other individual are solidly backfilled, there is no way that a new connection or link can be created.

Once the links and their ability to reconnect are removed, the healer can descend the frequencies by closing their chakras one by one from the seventh through to the first and return to the Earth level. Finish by offering the patient a glass of water to help ground them. The healer can also drink a glass of water to do the same.

Clearly this is only one method of visualizing the

link between two incarnate individuals. Other methods can be created and personalized according to the working practices and imagination of the healer to achieve the same thing.

Common links created in the current incarnation that influence the patient can be based upon the following overall themes:

- Control
- Coercion
- Subtle influence
- Inappropriate friendship
- Appropriate friendship
- Authority
- Responsibility
- Inappropriate support
- Appropriate support
- Addiction
- Subversion
- Betrayal
- Loyalty
- Comfort
- Empathy
- Love

With the plethora of ways in which links with others can affect us in this incarnation, should we let them, it is not surprising that many psychological (psycho-spiritual) issues we face are created as a function of them.

# Psychological Issues as a Function of a Higher Frequency Incarnation

## Attention Deficit Hyperactive Disorder (ADHD) and Attention Deficit Disorder (ADD)

ADHD is becoming more and more common and many medical professionals are associating it with a psychological disorder that can be associated with the patient's genome as a function of inheritance from parents or brain function/structure or chemical imbalance.

From a genetic perspective, although ADHD can run in the family it cannot, as yet, be attributable to a single gene or genetic fault and, as such, is likely to be complicated and is therefore not a robust answer to how it manifests. If we consider the brain, its structure and function the research findings have identified that there are a possible number of differences between those with and without ADHD but whether this can be classified as significant cannot be clarified. Supported theories suggest that certain areas of the brain may be smaller or larger in people with ADHD in comparison with those without. Other research goes on to suggest that those with ADHD could have an imbalance in the level of neurotransmitters in the brain, or that these chemicals are dysfunctional.

The symptoms of ADHD can be categorized into two **types of behavioral problems: inattentiveness and hyperactivity** and impulsiveness, although some patients cannot be classified as such (for more information, see https://www.nhs.uk/conditions/attention-deficit-hyperactivity-disorder-adhd/symptoms/). For example, patients with attention deficit disorder (ADD) can present inattentiveness, but not hyperactivity or impulsiveness. Because the symptoms may be less obvious, ADD can sometimes go unnoticed.

Both children and adults can have ADHD or ADD, although it can be argued that adult ADHD was undiagnosed when the adult patient was a child and therefore should not be age relative!

From the spiritual perspective, the healer may be presented with a child (or adult) as a patient that is difficult to control or get any long-term interest from in any subject, while the adult, as a patient, is usually considered as being bipolar.

The UK National Health Service (UK NHS) suggest that symptoms of ADHD in children and teenagers (young adults) are well defined, and they're usually noticeable before the age of six. They occur in more than one situation, such as at home and at school.

## Symptoms in Children

### Inattentiveness

The main signs of inattentiveness can be categorized as having a short attention span and being easily distracted; making careless mistakes, appearing forgetful, or losing things; lack of tolerance for tedious or time-consuming tasks, being unable to listen to or carry out instructions, or having difficulty in organizing tasks and/or constantly changing activity or task.

### Hyperactivity and Impulsiveness

The main signs of hyperactivity and impulsiveness can be categorized as being unable to sit still and therefore displaying constant fidgeting (excessive physical movement); inability to concentrate on tasks; excessive talking or interrupting conversations; impatience, inability to wait their turn; acting without thinking; and displaying little or no sense of danger.

These psycho-physical symptoms can cause significant problems in a child's life resulting in underachievement, poor social interaction with their peer group/adults, and resistance to discipline.

Although not always the case, some children may also have signs of other problems or conditions alongside ADHD such as anxiety, defiance, poor personal conduct, depression, levels of autism, epilepsy, and learning difficulties such as reading, writing, and understanding.

## Symptoms in Adults

ADHD symptoms are more difficult to define in adults, largely due to a lack of research. However, it is reasonable to assume that as a developmental disorder, an adult will have had ADHD as a child, which may not have been diagnosed. Other conditions such as depression, anxiety, or dyslexia may therefore continue through childhood, adolescence, and adulthood.

Although the symptoms applied to children can sometimes be applied to adults that potentially display ADHD, some specialists suggest that these symptoms can affect adults in a very different way, such as being subtler. This is because hyperactivity can decrease in adults while inattentiveness can increase with the pressures of adult life and responsibilities.

Some symptoms associated with adult ADHD can be classified as carelessness or poor attention to detail; inability to finish a task, but happily starts a new one; little or no organizational/prioritization skills; inability to focus; losing things or being forgetful; edginess and restlessness; talking out of turn; can't keep quiet, interrupting others; mood swings, irritability, quick to anger; inability to deal with stress, extreme impatience, and taking risks.

ADHD in adults can also occur alongside several related issues, problems, or conditions. Although the most common is depression, an adult with ADHD may also display personality, bipolar, and/or obsessive-compulsive disorders. As with children, adult ADHD creates behavioral problems such as difficulties with social interaction and creation and maintenance of relationships.

## The Spiritual/Energetic Explanation for ADHD, ADD, and Bipolarism

Presently there are a high number of "higher frequency" incarnate Aspects (Souls) on the Earth as more Aspects or Souls elect to incarnate to help in raising the overall frequency of the incarnate population and the Earth itself. This is to assist in the ability of the genre of Aspects that are classified as incarnate mankind to ascend into the next frequency of incarnate existence and compensate for the lower frequencies of another genre of incarnate Aspect. This other genre of incarnate Aspect is being used to "backfill" for those that ascend to the next frequency in their current incarnation and hence maintain the overall population, but that have a lower level quality of sentience to those that ascend. I classify them as backfill people because of the role they play. Their quality of sentience or sentient volume/mass is lower than the Aspects that normally incarnate in the Earth-based human form but is higher than those of the animal Aspects. They have only been allowed to incarnate on Earth and experience individualized free will in the past fifty to sixty years.

Many of these higher frequency incarnate Aspects have little or no experience in incarnating in this low frequency environment and therefore struggle. They are classified as Rainbow, Indigo, or Crystal Children and their hybrid states of incarnate frequency which are Rainbow/Indigo, Rainbow/Crystal, Indigo/Crystal, and Rainbow/Indigo/Crystal. Dolores Cannon further classified these children as "The Volunteers," of which there are three waves, each wave being attributable to a classification of higher frequency child. A later "fourth" wave, for the hybrids, was discovered and classified by the author. A further "fifth" wave limited to twelve "white" children whose role is based upon qualitative, quantitative, and "behind the scenes" spiritual "leading the leaders" leadership was also discovered by the author in 2014 when in China.

All of these children, many now adults, came and come into this incarnation with significantly higher levels of energetic communicative ability than their normal frequency incarnate Aspect counterparts, and so have an expectation to be able to communicate on many levels above and beyond the normal communication modalities of speech, writing, and body language. They often display autistic and savant qualities and so their cognitive abilities are significantly higher. Try to think of these people as trying to communicate with people energetically, telepathically, and telempathically (and many other unknown energetic communicative mediums) but with most people ignoring them because they aren't operating on these communicative levels. From a technical perspective it is like you, dear reader, trying to communicate via a video telephone with someone who is only able to use Morse code and a telegraph. The technologies are so different that they are totally incompatible. You as the person trying to communicate with the video telephone would get bored, frustrated, and impatient (maybe even angry, specifically if you expect the reciprocation of equal levels of communication) while the Morse code and telegraph user would be unaware or even oblivious of your attempts to communicate with them.

ADHD and ADD (and maybe other designations classified, or as yet not) are, in my experience, physical manifestations of boredom, frustration, and anger due to the lack of high frequency connectivity with others of the same or similar frequency as the patient who displays ADHD or ADD. As described above they subconsciously and naturally expect to be able to communicate on a higher level/s with everyone else around them and when they get no response they get frustrated and angry. Don't "we" get angry or frustrated when we are ignored? This is especially true of younger incarnates that have no understanding or concept of why they feel that they are being ignored. In essence, they are high-functioning individuals and need high frequency communicative mental stimulation as a result, but sadly are surrounded by low-functioning individuals and get no high frequency communicative mental stimulation.

With no other diagnosis available to medical and psychological professionals (that they are prepared to accept at this moment in time), many of these "high frequency" incarnates diagnosed as described above end up being on some form of medication to "calm them down" so that they behave like so-called "normal people" and don't get so agitated, frustrated, and/or angry. This appears to be consistent in most countries in the world.

The reason why the medication "appears to work" is because it creates a low frequency condition within the patient's physical and energetic bodies because of the disharmonious effect of the medication with the naturally higher frequencies for these individual's bodies. Anything that is not a natural occurring substance with in the body causes the potential for dysfunction and a reduction in frequency. Therefore, excessive use of alcohol, smoking products, and social drugs make us age faster and/or slower in thinking or being physically inactive. They can also affect the metabolism in other ways such as making us susceptible to virus or disease in a way that we would not be if we were "clean," so to speak.

Many people that I have worked with that are on prescribed medication for hyperactivity or bipolarism or that have been diagnosed as having ADHD have stated that the medication makes them feel heavy and slow and unable to think correctly, at least not in the way that they would want to or would normally think.

In real terms, there is no energy-based healing that would be effective for these patients because the medication is trying to supress their natural incarnate condition. In fact, the medication is not curing the issue either. Indeed, it is creating a condition where, to supposedly interact with society in the way that most of society expect them to interact or communicate with, they need to be on medication. Based upon this, the medication is creating a condition, a dependency, in order to integrate with others in an acceptable way, rather than solving the problem.

I don't condone the use of drugs to assist in high frequency functionality because it is a mechanical and temporary fix for something that is natural for the patient. It ultimately results in lack of health in the medium to long term and perpetuates a depressed state of beingness.

So, if they are functioning normally with reference to their own frequential state then there is no cure to be had. But if there is no cure available, then how can the healer help such high frequency individuals?

In my experience dealing with the parents of such children and their adult counterparts, the answer is two-fold. This is, provided the healer, through scanning the patient with the combined functionality of their intuition, spiritual/third eye, and visualization, can confirm that the patient's ADHD is a function of a higher frequency existence with little or no communication with others rather than a chemical imbalance of some sort.

**First:** the patient normally benefits in being advised why they are being classified as having ADHD from the spiritual perspective. In this way the healer needs to advise the patient of the different classifications of "children" (Rainbow, Crystal, Indigo—see above), their reasons for incarnation and that they will be communicating on many channels subconsciously while expecting responses from these subconscious communications and not actually getting them, in most instances. The healer also needs to advise the child, or adult, that their parents may not be able to communicate with them. Within this, the healer needs to ask some key questions from the patient about how they feel or perceive things in order to satisfy themselves that they are dealing with ADHD as a result of higher frequency existence with limited, or no, communication on the same level.

Nonexhaustive examples of these questions are:

- Do you feel that you were ignored as a child? (for adults)
- Do you feel that you are ignored (now) [adult or child]?
- Do you have trouble getting all your words out?
- Do you feel that your mind is full and that you can't speak fast enough to get everything out?
- Do you feel like you can do everything at once?
- Did you stutter (as a child or now)?
- Do you feel that people don't listen to you?
- Do you feel like you are from somewhere else?
- Do you get frustrated with people don't do what you want them to do without telling them verbally?
- Do you feel that people should understand your thoughts?
- Do you feel that people should know what you want?
- Do you feel that speaking is too slow?
- Do you use intuition a lot?
- Do you get answers to your questions in your mind before you have the actual "worked out and therefore logical" answer?
- Are there people around you who you feel know what you are thinking without verbally communicating with them? Do these people also have ADHD? Are there many of these

people? Can you gain access to them?

- Do you feel you have higher levels of communicative functionality normally available to you?

In the event that the patient answers positively (yes) to over 75 percent of these questions, in my experience a person with ADHD will say yes to all of them, then you will be able to work with them from the spiritual perspective. Getting the answers to the questions above will set the scene for the second part.

**Second:** work with the child's parents (or the patient themselves if they are adults) to understand where other children (or adults) can be found who also have ADHD. In my experience putting children (or adults) who display ADHD together in the same space, goes a long way to solving the problem and creating a healing condition for them. This is because they are "at long last" able to communicate with someone on the same level as themselves.

Frustration can be lifted (especially if on medication) by performing the chakra opening exercises (described previously for use by the healer to move to the correct frequency level, but can be used by the patient for therapeutic purposes) as it will help to lift the frequencies of the patient. It will create a higher level of understanding of their environment and those whom they interact with within their environment due to maintaining a higher level of communicative functionality therefore reducing the frustration (ADHD) in the process.

The child (or adult) needs to be told that even those they love the most, and who love them the most, their parents, are most likely not of the same frequency as they are and therefore are not able to communicate with them in the way that they expect or require.

In essence, in this second part, and linked in with the details from the first part, the healer takes on board the role of spiritual counselor. This is because the child, their parent/s, or the adult will need "direction" or guidance for a period of time to assist in the child's or adult's continued understanding and acceptance of self and the limitations of those around them. This in itself will form the basis of a robust healing process culminating with successful integration into so-called "normal" society while integrating with a higher frequency society.

### Bipolarism

It is quite common for an incarnate human vehicle to have more than one Aspect (Soul) associated with it. Usually only one Aspect is allowed to be the primary Aspect. This means that they are the only Aspect (Soul) that is supposed to be able to animate the human vehicle and interact with others within its environment. Bipolarism is usually a function of two Aspects associated with the incarnate human vehicle who alternate command and control of the human vehicle. More often than not they have a different "personality" and level of emotional interaction/expression or temper.

The cure for this is a function of psycho-spiritual healing where the primary incarnating Aspect is reassigned as such with the secondary Aspect being permanently placed in a position of passive observation (compartmentalization), without being able to interact with the primary Aspect. For details on how to compartmentalize one or more Aspects and reassign command and control of the incarnate human vehicle to the primary Aspect, please see the section on this subject called "Compartmentalizing or Reassignation of Control" below.

# Client Specific or "Bespoke" Healing

Client specific or "bespoke" healing is not the simple administration of certain healing techniques, such as chelation or spine cleansing as a one-size-fits-all healing process. These are specific healing techniques designed to heal specific issues. In the two examples cited, that would be basic energy balancing and realignment of the energies of the spine, administered either at the request of the patient or the healer gaining information in one of the ways below that results in the need for a generalized or specific healing. For instance, Reiki is a generalized low-level general healing modality, whereas astral entity removal is specific to removing an astral entity and EFT (Emotional Freedom Technique) is specialized in removing emotional blockages.

Client specific or bespoke healing is then, by definition, what most advanced healers give to their patients. That being, the healer gains information about the patient, analyzes the information and administers a healing regime appropriate to their findings. The healing regime is based upon guided and intuitive information resulting in a mixture of the components of different healing modalities performed together within a single healing appointment to affect a holistic healing regime for a specific client with one or several issues.

Administering a general modality when a specific modality is necessary, and vice versa, does not affect a robust healing. Additionally, administering a specific or generalized healing when a bespoke healing is required also does not affect a robust healing.

Understanding if the patient requires a bespoke healing and what the content of the bespoke healing will be is achieved by the following:

1. Asking questions to decide physical issues.
2. Asking questions to decide psychological issues (psycho-spiritual).
3. Asking the patient's guide.
4. Asking the healer's guide.
5. Information gained from energetically scanning the patient with their third eye or intuitive vision. Looking at the energy system (energy templates, chakras, and auric layers) of the patient. Also included is looking for the presence of astral entities.
6. Observing the patient's body language (signs of nervousness, frustration, indecision, over- or underemphasis/enthusiasm for certain issues/subjects, fear, over- or under-confidence).
7. Observing the patient's physical demeanor (physical health).
8. Observing the patient's psychological demeanor (mental health).
9. Establishing the links between the physical, psychological, and energetic aspects of the patient to establish the root cause of the physical or psychological issues to be healed.

By asking the questions and making the observations above, and establishing the links between them, the healer can create a psycho-spiritual and physio-spiritual profile for the patient.

Please note that this "bespoke" profile may only be useful for one healing appointment. However, some aspects of it may be useful in additional appointments if necessary. Also note that as the number of patients increases, the healer may notice that certain combinations of "bespoke" healing components can be reused on other patients.

Although a healing modality may be needed in totality with one patient, the components (the "smaller" aspects of a healing modality) may be singled out. This means that only the components necessary (the useful or necessary smaller aspects of a healing modality extracted from an overall healing modality) to affect a robust healing should be used.

There is no point, or need to, administer a full body energy template healing on seven frequency levels when only the energy templates of, for example, a spleen, are required.

Similarly, there is no need to ask the patient to come back for five appointments to administer a "full" chelation, spine cleanse, chakra repair, astral entity removal, or energy template repair/replacement when the healing can be administered by a competent healer in one appointment by extracting only those components from a chelation, spine cleansing, chakra repair, astral entity removal, or energy template replacement/replacements that are necessary.

It is the role of the healer to get the patient back to health as quickly and as robustly as possible and not to drag out the healing process over a number of weeks or months, which sometimes happens, for "financial" reasons!

Remember the healing must be efficient and robust while being time and cost effective.

Although, this book only deals with the healing modalities that I have been taught, have used, and have been given to me by The Source to help my patients when the healing modalities I had were not effective or available, one should not rule out the use of the components of other healing modalities that you as the healer may have, but that are not mentioned in this text.

Below are a few of the combinations of components, multi-mixed and single, of the healing modalities I have used with my patients. This is by no means an exhaustive list and is continuously growing in both diversity and complexity.

- Full chelation, all chakras cleaned, psycho-spiritual reprogramming (anxiety, confidence, fear)
- Specific chakra reconstruction and/or replacement
- Chelation on the lower body, energy template repair on all templates on the lower body
- Energy template repair on a major organ
- Astral entity removal, full chelation, full chakra clean/repair, repair of energy templates and human energy field (auric layers) where astral entity has connected to the patient
- Energetically replace the energy templates associated with the endocrine system
- Energetically replace the energy templates associated with the nervous system
- Full chelation, introduction of a psychic shield
- Full chelation, full spinal cleanse
- Energetically replace the energy templates associated with a patient's knee
- Energy realignment of the vertebrae in the lumbar region (only), psycho-spiritual reprogramming (standing up for one's self)
- Full chelation, DNA reprogramming (described below) to stop ovarian cyst growth, replacement of energy templates of the ovaries to templates that don't support ovarian cyst growth
- Replacement of the energy templates of the

heart, repair the energy templates of the lungs

- Removal of astral mucus, repair of the human energy field (auric layers) where the astral mucus had woven itself in to the auric layers
- Full chelation, removal of karmic links to another incarnate aspect (soul), psycho-spiritual reprogramming (remove negative feelings and responses to the incarnate aspect [soul] connected to the patient via karma)
- Removal of past life links, removal of energy associated with the method of demise experienced in that past life. For example, the links are removed from an incarnation that terminated by drowning, psycho-spiritual reprogramming to remove a fear of water will be necessary.
- Chakra cleanse
- Full chelation

In essence, the number of combinations of healing modality components that the healer can use is infinite. The only limitation is the lack of expansivity of the healer themselves.

# Psycho-Spiritual Reprogramming

Psycho-spiritual reprogramming is a healing modality that was given to me by The Source.

In my experience, it is an extremely effective alternative healing process to psychotherapy and/or medication to bring a patient's perceptions, deep-rooted psychological issues, thoughts, behaviors, and actions into order. That being, those that create problems in the way the patient interacts with those around them and the environment within which they exist. Some or most of the psychological conditions can and do create habits and their physical and mental manifestations. A few of the basic psychological functions that need healing or correcting are fears, anxiety, confidence, preconceptions or beliefs, expectations, and habits.

Many of the psychological functions above can be generically represented by the term "schizophrenia" (that being, at some level or progressing toward), which according to many mental health institutions is classified as a long-term mental disorder and that this mental disorder involves a breakdown in the relationship between thought, emotion, and behavior. Schizophrenia therefore leads to faulty perception, inappropriate actions and feelings, withdrawal from reality, and personal relationships, moving the patient into fantasy and/or delusion together with a level of mental fragmentation.

Schizophrenia can also be subcategorized as being paranoid, disorganized, catatonic, childhood, and schizoaffective disorders. The reader is encouraged to undertake some personal research to further understand these descriptions and the suggested reasons for them. However, irrespective of the accepted medical descriptions afforded to the subcategories above, most modalities of schizophrenia can lead to psychosis. Psychosis is classified as a severe mental disorder in which thought and emotions are so impaired that contact is lost with external reality. In metaphysical terms this means the reality within which we accept as the current reality. From the nonmetaphysical perspective, it means that they have difficulty in relating to that which happens around them, that which the general populous calls reality.

It is clear that, whichever modality of healing or treatment is used, the individual displaying schizophrenic tendencies declines in their interactive abilities and is well on their way to becoming psychotic if not treated or healed. The usual signs that are displayed by a schizophrenic or psychotic patient are a drop in personal performance, inability to think in a clear way, lack of trust, poor personal grooming or hygiene, preferring to be alone or displaying extreme, inappropriate feelings or even no emotions at all.

Those patients who have displayed some or all of the symptoms above have usually had an experience that has either been passed over from a previous incarnation, or they have had an experience in this current incarnation that has affected them in a profound way.

Such experiences can be:

- Method of demise (past incarnation)
- Betrayal (past or current incarnation)
- Trauma (past or current incarnation)
    - Physical abuse
    - Sexual abuse
    - Mental abuse
    - Being controlled
    - Slavery
    - Abduction

    - Accident
    - Illness
    - Bullying
    - Being ignored
    - Being used
- Inappropriate expectations of personal performance
    - What the patient thinks they should be able to do
    - What the patient thinks others (usually authority figures) think they should be able to do

The most common manifestations of the experiences above, which lead to schizophrenia, bipolar disorder, and psychosis, are:

Mental

- Depression
- Lack of self-worth
- Anxiety
- Lack of confidence
- Addiction (drugs, alcohol, sensory stimulus, including self-harm)
- Lack of trust

Physical

- Knee problems
- Back problems
- Low energy
- Poor eyesight
- Poor circulation
- Impaired heart function or tightness of chest

Psycho-spiritual reprogramming seeks to change the way the patient thinks, behaves, and acts by changing their mental state. This means changing the psychological programming that allows the patient to continue to think, behave, and act inappropriately or relatively to their environment. It also allows the healer to change the physical manifestations (diseases or illnesses) associated with chronic psychological conditions because in most cases the energetic templates of the incarnate human vehicle adopt the disharmonious frequencies of the abnormal thoughts, behaviors, and actions resulting in the gross physical aspect of the incarnate human vehicle following the new programming of the energetic templates resulting from disharmonious mental conditions.

In order to change these dysfunctional thoughts that result in dysfunctional behaviors and actions, and in some cases the physical manifestations of disease, illness, and restrictive movement, the healer needs to change the psycho-spiritual program at the root cause.

I have used many different ways to change this programming, ranging from talking the patient through the reasons for their psycho-spiritual condition through to meditating on the patient while conducting a healing resulting in my sitting in a deep and dark vault. This vault is full of old-fashioned eighteenth-century contact breaker types of switches, each representing part of their programming or "belief system," the total system representing the psycho-spiritual condition of the patient. The final and most efficient way that I have found is visualizing sitting at a computer terminal and entering into the diagnostics routine of that computer. The diagnostics, again, representing the psycho-spiritual condition of the patient.

Another function of psycho-spiritual programming is DNA reprogramming. This requires a different method of visualization and is, when appropriate, combined with my normal methods of psycho-spiritual healing to create an in-depth and robust response to some of the more aggressive physical manifestations of incorrect or inappropriate psycho-spiritual programming. DNA reprogramming will be explained in a chapter on its own.

## How to Perform Psyco-Spiritual Reprogramming

Due to the potential for changing the psychological responses of an individual in terms of how they interact with themselves, their environment, and those within their environment, I consider psycho-spiritual reprogramming to be a very advanced healing modality. As a result of this, I strongly suggest that only experienced individuals with a full-time practice of over five years in the service of being a healer should embark upon the use of the techniques that I am about to describe. Although they may appear to be simple, it is the ability to see beyond the obvious that allows this work to be successful in a most positive way and not just place a sticking plaster on the issue being experienced by the patient.

The psycho-spiritual reprogramming process that I find most useful is one where I place myself in the diagnostic routines of the psycho-spiritual programming of the patient.

In order to achieve this, I will have connected to the patient energetically as part of the usual consultation process. Within the consultation (see previous chapters that illustrate the questions that I normally use) I usually establish that there are a number of issues that affect the patient in a psycho-spiritual way, rather than physical, that is different from the normal past life or current life link either with themselves or another. These psycho-spiritual issues can either be psychological, psychological with a physiological response (dysfunction), or a physiological response caused by an incorrect DNA program. These are my main categories.

Typically, a patient may advise me that they feel uneasy in certain situations, with certain people or certain environments. For example, they feel anxious, stressed, depressed, unworthy, lacking in confidence, or are unable to articulate themselves properly. These feelings can sometimes be associated with some form of physiological response such as knee problems, back ache or problems, stomach problems, poor liver or kidney function, palpitations, sight issues, and poor circulation (*not an exhaustive list —GSN*). At other times the patient knows that they have a potentially terminal illness such as cancer, multiple sclerosis, fibromyalgia, or autoimmune diseases, which are all based upon some form of DNA dysfunction.

Once I have established that, as a result of the patient's verbal response to my questions and/or the information about the patient I have gained through connecting with them energetically, there is a psycho-spiritual issue, I categorize it as stated above as either psychological, psychological with physiological response, or DNA mis-programming.

Psycho-spiritual reprogramming can be achieved with equal success during a hands-on physical healing at the clinic of the healer or via distance healing because it is an energetic healing modality that works on the psycho-spiritual aspects of the energetic templates that create the incarnate human vehicle.

Wherever the patient is located I seek their permission to reprogram them, even if they already agree to a healing, such is the potential impact on the patient.

I will first describe a general process that I use before further describing the more specific processes for the primary issues surrounding psychological, psychological with physiological responses, or DNA mis-programming; I will use examples later on in this chapter that are based upon my own experience.

With the patient lying or sitting in a comfortable position, the healer closes their eyes and focuses their closed eye vision on the location of the spiritual or third eye, which is in between the eyebrows and above the bridge of the nose. Next the healer should meditate on the patient, focusing their consciousness on becoming one with the energies of the patient from a psycho-spiritual perspective. In order to do this, I see myself as being inside the patient and moving down into the very center of the essence of the incarnate Aspect or soul, at the Soul Seat, that point where the sentience of the Aspect resides during incarnation. The Soul Seat is positioned behind the front aspect of the heart chakra.

Once my sentience is positioned in the same location as the Soul Seat I then ask to see the psycho-spiritual programming of the patient presented to me as if I was at a computer terminal. Furthermore, I ask to see the detail behind the programming in terms of looking at a diagnostic routine or list of diagnostic settings with each aspect of the patient's psycho-spiritual response as a tick box that is either "ON" or "OFF." I then change the state of the individual settings from "ON" to "OFF" or "OFF" to "ON" or leave them alone as necessary. For instance, one would turn anxiety "OFF" but confidence "ON."

Similar or deeper layers of diversification are normally seen in people who display psychological issues such as anxiety, for example, because there may be a number of issues that cause anxiety and some of them may have deeper layers associated with them, such as a certain person in a certain environment with certain other people discussing a certain subject that always comes up that causes anxiety within the patient and ultimately fear about experiencing this situation again or on a regular basis. Although one can work with reprogramming the top layer or "general" topic that needs to be healed, it is just that, a generalized reprogramming and will not work robustly on specific issues. The diagnostic settings, shown with three layers of diversification, can be visualized as shown below:

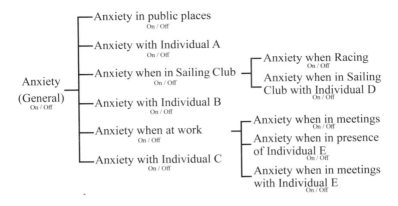

- Anxiety (General) On / Off
  - Anxiety in public places On / Off
  - Anxiety with Individual A On / Off
  - Anxiety when in Sailing Club On / Off
    - Anxiety when Racing On / Off
    - Anxiety when in Sailing Club with Individual D On / Off
  - Anxiety with Individual B On / Off
  - Anxiety when at work On / Off
    - Anxiety when in meetings On / Off
    - Anxiety when in presence of Individual E On / Off
    - Anxiety when in meetings with Individual E On / Off
  - Anxiety with Individual C On / Off

In terms of confidence, or lack of it, as an issue that needs psycho-spiritual reprogramming the healer needs to add diversified layers together by turning "ON" all layers affected to ensure that the full application of confidence is available to the patient, and not just being confident in, say, riding a bicycle but is limited in, or has low, confidence in anything else they do.

However …

When I work on confidence levels within the layer I also add another function. This function is the ability of the healer to not just turn "ON" or "OFF" confidence, but to turn it "UP" or "DOWN." This allows overconfidence to be dealt with without creating a condition where turning "OFF" the confidence in the area of overconfidence affecting or connected to other layers of confidence that are required to be "ON" causes new issues. It also allows the healer to turn "UP" areas of confidence without affecting areas of connected confidence that need to remain "LOW" or nearly "OFF."

In the illustration below, based upon cancer, I have again shown three layers of diversification. The diversification is focused on breast cancer as an example. However, it should also be noted that this is only the psycho-spiritual predisposition to cancer and not therapy via DNA reprogramming; both modalities of healing may be necessary. A general reprogramming is sufficient if the healer is dealing with changing a disposition to any cancer but if the patient is experiencing one of the types of cancer in a lower layer then the type in the lower layer needs to be the specific target for the psycho-spiritual reprogramming. Additionally, this may and usually does, need to be augmented by the use of DNA reprogramming as well.

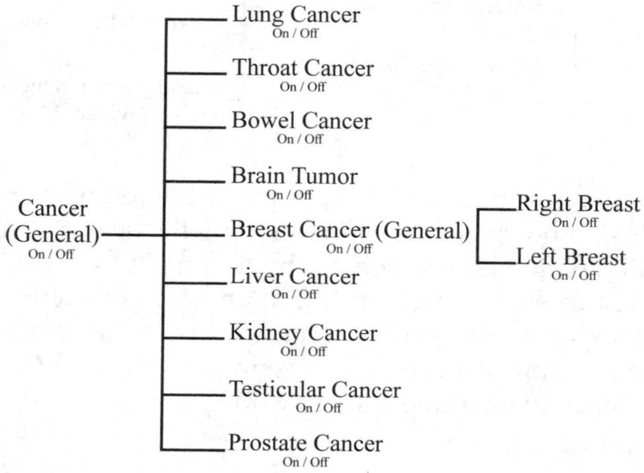


Once I have selected the correct sequence of "ON" and "OFF" and/or "UP" (increased) or "DOWN" (decreased) layers and parameters within these layers I then need to assign these settings to the seven templates that create the incarnate human vehicle.

I do this by again assigning an "ON"/"OFF" tick box to the energetic template that I am assigning the psycho-spiritual programming to. I select "ON" to all of the energetic templates and the frequency levels that they are associated with.

Why do I assign the psycho-spiritual programming to all seven energetic templates? The answer is this. Whereas one can heal an organ or a chakra on a specific energy template or number of energy templates for specific healings, psycho-spiritual healing needs to be applied to all seven energy templates because it needs to affect the whole incarnate human vehicle. A chakra, for example, only needs to be healed on the frequency level and energetic template that it is predominantly represented on and by. An organ, other body part, or even the whole body can be healed on all seven energy templates or just one or more from a psycho-spiritual perspective. This is because psycho-spiritual issues can start at lower frequency levels than the seventh and above.

For example, a physical ailment can require the gross physical energy templates to be healed (the first three frequencies and energy templates) but the psycho-spiritual issue/s that caused the physical dysfunction/disease to manifest may only be prominent on the fourth and/or fifth frequency level, the astral level, and/or the etheric template. Based upon this, work on the sixth and seventh frequencies and energy templates is not required because the psycho-spiritual issues do not exist there (feel free to check, though). An example of my tick boxes seen in the psycho-spiritual programming of a patient is below.

| | | |
|---|---|---|
| 1st Frequency Level | Etheric Body | On/Off |
| 2nd Frequency Level | Emotional Layer | On/Off |
| 3rd Frequency Level | Mental Body | On/Off |
| 4th Frequency Level | Astral Level | On/Off |
| 5th Frequency Level | Etheric Template | On/Off |
| 6th Frequency Level | Celestial Body | On/Off |
| 7th Frequency Level | Ketheric Template | On/Off |

Once I have ticked "ON" to all of the energetic templates and their subsequent frequency levels that I want the psycho-spiritual reprogramming to be affective on, I then visualize a tick box that has the function of an overall "SAVE" function. This finalizes the overall reprogramming of the psycho-spiritual aspects of the patient that needed to be corrected.

What I have described above is an example of the process from a high-level perspective. In the three examples to follow I will describe a particular condition for each of the genres of psycho-spiritual reprogramming that I have encountered. I have no doubt that there are other genres but to date I have not personally experienced them or been advised of any from other healers I know.

## Psychological

Psychological issues are the predominant reason for using psycho-spiritual reprogramming and the main reason that I use this modality.

I usually find that the main basis for psychological issues within a patient revolve around depression, anxiety, and confidence and that these are a downstream function of some event that the patient has experienced early on in their lives. Mental or physical abuses by a relative, parent, or trusted friend are high up on the list of causes. Depression, anxiety, and confidence are the very high-level conditions that can be relative to either overall states of being or states of being that are focused upon the patient experiencing certain environments, individuals, or individuals within certain environments and certain levels of interaction. Don't forget to refer to the deeper levels of psychosis mentioned in a previous chapter on this subject.

In this example, I will deal with confidence relative to communicating during business or other meetings of people. Although confidence can be turned up or down, it first needs to be turned "ON" relative to the personal interactive situations where the patient experiences reduced levels of confidence.

Ask the patient to sit down or lie down comfortably on a therapy bed or suitable couch. Ask them to relax. Close your own eyes and change your focus to the location of the spiritual or third eye, which is in between the eyebrows and above the bridge of the nose. With the patient's permission meditate on being connected to them. Next, change the focus of your sentience away from the third eye and into the location of the Soul Seat, which is behind the origin of the front aspect of the heart chakra (see Barbara Brennan's book *Hands of Light* for further information).

Visualize sitting down in a room that has a computer terminal and that this computer terminal allows you access to the psycho-spiritual program associated with the patient. Using your mental voice ask the patient to show you the programming associated with confidence. As with the examples above you will see a hierarchy, like an organizational structure or family tree that identifies a list of things that the patient associates with being confident, including the overall subject of confidence "in general." Look down the list to see where there is a lack of confidence associated with being in meetings, business or otherwise. When you see the area of concern you may see that confidence in meetings has a number of components to it, such as attending meetings in general is OK but attending meetings that are to feed back a certain type of information to a certain individual are the main focus of lack of confidence in meetings.

Trace the line from the main focus of the lack of confidence back up the hierarchical structure, the family tree of confidence, to the highest point that is the general subject of confidence within the programming of the patient. Assign tick boxes or "ON"/"OFF" boxes to each of the areas of confidence that join together from the focus of the lack of confidence through to the overall subject heading of general confidence. Tick them all as "ON." Now assign a method of increasing the confidence at the focus of the lack of confidence and those related issues that are on the line between the focus and the general confidence heading and that are within the next two layers above the main focus. That method of increasing the confidence can be like a volume control on a radio or television where turning the control clockwise increases the confidence and turning the control counterclockwise reduces the confidence. Turn controls to the right until you feel that they represent 85 percent of the total level of confidence available. (It's always best to have some in reserve!) Now visualize a tick box that says "LOCK"; this is to lock the control at that level. Visualize the "LOCK" being "ON" for all of the areas of confidence that have had controls assigned to them.

Once you have increased the confidence levels in those areas that relate to and are the main focus of the lack of confidence in meetings, you need to tick "ON" to all of the energetic templates and their subsequent frequency levels that you want the psycho-spiritual reprogramming relative to confidence to be affective on. Finally, visualize a tick box that has the function of an overall "SAVE" function. This finalizes the overall reprogramming of the psycho-spiritual aspects of the patient that needed to be corrected to allow them to be confident in meetings where they expressed a lack of or limited levels of confidence.

Please note that in extreme cases this may need to be repeated a small number of times. With one patient who experienced extreme anxiety in public places I gave around four minor "Top-Up's" as and when requested before a complete cure was experienced. Also note that this particular patient had tried various forms of psychotherapy and medication prior to this healing.

## Psychological with Physiological Response

Simply put, a client who displays both a physiological and a psychological issue or issues will need to have both conditions healed during the same consultation period. This is because they will be linked together; that being, the physical issue will be a manifestation of the psychological issue in some way, shape, or form.

For example, the following psycho-spiritual and physiological conditions are linked together. Please note, however, that this is in no way an exhaustive list.

| Psycho-Spiritual Issues | Physiological Issues | Potential Healing Modality |
|---|---|---|
| Poor Confidence | Back Issues | Psycho-Spiritual reprogramming for confidence (pride, standing straight), repair (reconstruct), rebuild, replace energy template for the back, perform spine cleansing. |
| Poor Confidence | Knee Problems | Psycho-Spiritual reprogramming for confidence (standing up for oneself, motivation). Repair (reconstruct), rebuild, replace energy template for the affected knee/knees, entire leg. |
| Anxiety (Surrounding a Certain Circumstance) | Stomach / Bowel Issues | Psycho-Spiritual reprogramming for anxiety (confidence, trust in oneself and one's ability). Repair (reconstruct), rebuild, replace energy template for the upper and lower stomach, bowels, oesophagus. |
| Anxiety (Surrounding interacting with a known person or persons) | Stomach / Bowel Issues, back, knee, or leg issues | Psycho-Spiritual reprogramming for anxiety (confidence, trust in oneself and one's ability or standing up for oneself, motivation). Repair (reconstruct), rebuild, replace energy template for the upper and lower stomach, bowels, esophagus. Repair (reconstruct), rebuild, replace energy template for the affected knee/knees, entire leg. |

| | | |
|---|---|---|
| Anxiety (about one's physical condition), can be associated with depression | Overall appearance, weight, beauty, sex | Psycho-Spiritual reprogramming for anxiety (acceptance of oneself, abilities, motivation to change one's physical appearance). Reconstruct, replace energy template for the total body, if necessary. |
| Self-Loathing (negative comparison wih others), can be depression as well | Overall appearance, weight, beauty, sex | Psycho-Spiritual reprogramming for self-comparison (acceptance of oneself, abilities, motivation to change one's physical appearance). Reconstruct, replace energy template for the total body, if necessary. |
| Self-Loathing (self-harm) | Overall appearance, weight, beauty, sex | Psycho-Spiritual reprogramming for anxiety (acceptance of oneself, preference of oneself without harming oneself). Reconstruct, replace energy template for the total body, if necessary. |
| Fear/Dread of animals/insects | Bite wounds, attack wounds, past (life?) memory | Psycho-Spiritual reprogramming for fear (turn off fear in "general" and for the specific animal, insect interaction). Reconstruct energy template for the affected body part, if necessary. |
| Dislike of certain foodstuffs (forced to eat certain foods) | Illness, abhorrent taste, food poisoning, sickness, and diarrhea. Allergies (ask the potient to check with their medical professional as well) | Psycho-Spiritual reprogramming for dislike (turn off dislike in "general" and for the specific foodstuff the patient dislikes). Turn off allergic reactions in "general" and with certain food stuffs. Reconstruct energy template for the digestive system, if necessary. Reprogram or replace the autoimmune system. |

In the instance that a client needs to be healed both psychologically and physiologically then the healer will need to administer a healing that incorporates a level of psycho-spiritual reprogramming, organ or body part reconstruction, and maybe an energetic template reconstruction. In the instance of a back problem then the healer will also need to perform a spine cleansing. Indeed, it is quite possible that other healing modalities may also need to be incorporated such as astral entity removal, foreign object removal, or auric layer reconstruction/repair. In any event or combination of healing modalities the healer needs to decide the most urgent task or tasks to perform and perform it/them in order of priority while they have the patient in their consultation room, including deciding if they need additional visits.

Having previously described the process surrounding an organ or body part reconstruction via the appropriate energy template/s earlier on in this book, as well as the process surrounding a psycho-spiritual reprogramming above, I will not describe them again but will describe the order of healing modality when faced with such a patient.

In all the healing that I have performed I have found that if I changed the psycho-spiritual programming of the patient before reconstructing the affected body part, there was an element of resistance with the reconstruction. This is because the psycho-spiritual program was in variance with the energy template/s associated with the body part that required healing and that was dysfunctional. The program needs to work hand in hand with the template/s and will attempt to change the template/s rather than work with it/them. However, the template/s will be playing catchup and as a result will cause the patient to experience confusion and discomfort. It's a bit like running a new operating system on an old computer that has neither the memory capacity nor the processing power to allow the new program to run effectively. Based upon this, I always perform the healing modality first and the psycho-spiritual reprogramming second. In this way, the energy templates of the newly reconstructed body part or organ are functional, but inert, until the psycho-spiritual programming has been applied.

Clearly not every organ or body part reconstruction requires a psycho-spiritual program, but those where the body part or organs dysfunction is caused by a psychological issue or incorrect thought process, do. As a result, when the healer notes that there is a psycho-spiritual issue associated with an illness that requires the energy template to be reconstructed the healing process goes much smoother when the energy template/s are repaired/reconstructed first and the associated psycho-spiritual reprograming is performed second.

## Psycho-Spiritual and DNA Reprogramming

With psycho-spiritual reprogramming already described I will focus on the process of DNA reprogramming. First, though, it is worth noting that as with the order of work between psycho-spiritual programming and organ/body part reconstruction, psycho-spiritual reprogramming and DNA reprogramming also have to be performed in order to be successful. In this instance, DNA reprogramming also needs to be performed before psycho-spiritual reprogramming, and if there are energetic templates to be reconstructed as well, the DNA needs to be reprogrammed before the energetic templates, with the psycho-spiritual healing taking place last.

There is a reason for this, and I will explain it.When there is a link between the energetic templates and psycho-spiritual programming the psycho-spiritual program controls the energetic templates. The energetic templates are configured to work with the psycho-spiritual program, and there is no resistance or variance in the program versus what is expected of the program by the energetic templates. The energetic templates transmit via the energetic aspect of RNA what the gross physical aspect of the incarnate human form needs to perform. The energetic aspect of the program is applied to the DNA, which is already configured to work with the information it received from the RNA. This information is transmitted biochemically to cell proteins from the DNA via the physical aspect of the RNA to the cell protein. The cell protein, having been told what its physical function is responds to a biochemical check, that being the right cell with the right function and signature is in the right body part or organ and is not rejected. If the cell is not rejected by those cells of the greater body part or organ or the autoimmune system, then the cell responds with a biochemical message of acceptance (rather like a check sum in an algorithm) which is sent to the DNA via the RNA. Once this message is received, the DNA sends an energetic response via the energetic side of the RNA to the energy template, which records the correct application of the original template requirement within the template turning off any further requirements. In the event that there is a need to feedback concurrence of the correct application of the templates program to the psycho-spiritual program then this is done, and the patient will feel at ease, have a feeling of well-being, and experience good health.

DNA reprogramming is a remarkably effective healing modality that affects the gross physical aspect of the incarnate human vehicle in a dramatic way. It can reverse the effect of cancers, genetic disorders, and even the ageing process.

In order to reprogram the DNA, the healer should first know what aspect of the patient's DNA is dysfunctional by both verbal questioning, other healthcare professionals' reports, and by using their third eye (intuition) to scan the body of the patient to establish which genetic dysfunction they have and therefore what needs to be healed. Once the dysfunction has been identified the healer then uses their visualization to see the DNA strand where the dysfunction is located as the spiral ladder-like shape that is the popular image used to describe it.

Next unwind the DNA strand so that you see the DNA as a ladder. The dysfunctional aspect of the DNA, for example, ovarian cysts or multiple sclerosis, will be represented by one of the "rungs" on the ladder. Look for the "rung" that identifies itself with the dysfunction you are healing. Once you have established which rung creates the dysfunction you are working with use your energetic hands to "pluck" the rung out of the ladder of the DNA strand and place it in your recycling bin. This will leave a gap. Next, using your energetic hands pluck out the two "vertical" aspects of the DNA strand that attaches the lower rung to the rung that you have just removed. Now you have the DNA strand in two pieces, the gap being where the rung and vertical aspects of the DNA strand that were causing the dysfunction were removed. Use your energetic hands to bring the two halves of the DNA together, making the two halves one again. You have now removed the aspect of the DNA that was causing the illness or dysfunction and the gross physical aspects that are manifest as a result of the dysfunction. Finally use your energetic hands and intention to recoil the DNA so that it adopts the same natural shape that it had before your work on it. Now gently move out of the energies of the patient and suggest that they take a drink of water to ground them.

## Illustration of the Removal of DNA Rung and Reattachment of the Two Severed Strands

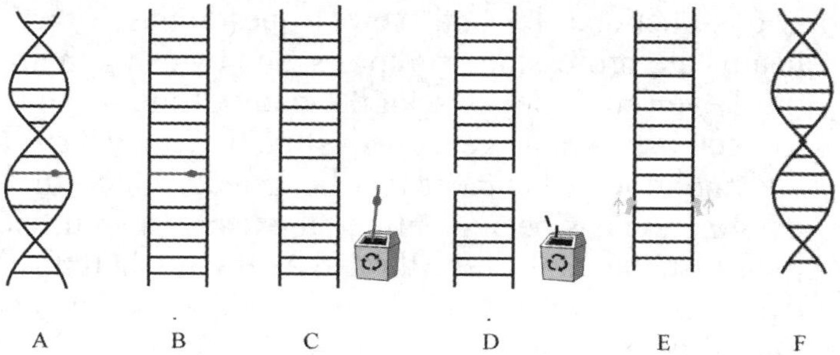

Provided that the patient or client is in tune with you as the healer and that they irrevocably "know" that they are healed, then the genetic dysfunctions will disappear very quickly. If, however, the patient or client has any doubt that they are healed—for instance, if they come to you after being seen by a long list of healers as a last attempt to be healed—then any microscopic amount of doubt will be enough to stop or reverse the healing process.

The healer also needs to note the following:

It is possible that the patient or client is not supposed to be healed, that they chose to experience the illness or disease as part of this incarnation, or that this disease or dysfunction is the method that they have chosen to terminate this incarnation—the disease, dysfunction, or illness being the method of their demise. If this is the case, your efforts to heal the patient will be to no avail.

# Dementia and Alzheimer's Disease

Physiologically, dementia and Alzheimer's disease are a function of the atrophy of the brain of the patient. Spiritually, dementia and Alzheimer's disease are a function of the incarnate aspect's desire to leave the current incarnation. The physiological function being a result of the spiritual it is therefore incurable from the physiological perspective because it is ultimately the result of the withdrawal of the sentience and associated energies of the incarnate aspect in a gradual way (with various speeds) from its current incarnation. Once the aspect has decided to leave an incarnation in this way there is generally no way to stop it because it is one of a number of ways in which an aspect detaches from an incarnation. An aspect only returns from a "near-death experience" if it is in their life plan to do so, such as a sudden and total remission from a usually terminal disease or the physical body has suffered significant and almost irretrievable damage in an accident of some sort, but that it is still useful to the aspect in terms of its ability to complete its life plan.

The only way in which dementia or Alzheimer's disease could be reversed is if the gradually departing aspect could be persuaded to return to its incarnation. However, because an aspect generally departs from its incarnation as a result of the life plan or the essence of the components of the life plan have been experienced in a full or acceptable way, this is not generally possible. When an aspect (soul) decides to, or has the opportunity to return home, it is more than happy to do so. This is why physiological attempts to restore the brain show minor success and then fail. Additionally, one needs to be reminded that the sentience of an aspect does not reside in the brain, but in the Soul Seat, and that this illustrates the fact that the brain is not a controlling reason for the cause of dementia or Alzheimer's but that it is a function of a slow disassociation of an aspect from its incarnate human vehicle. Incidentally, Parkinson's disease, in all of its variants, can be considered in a similar if not same way.

As a result, the text below, which is an abridged version of a lecture I gave on this subject during the May World Satsanga in 2019, is designed to offer a greater understanding of this subject and not a cure, whether it be physiological, energetic, or psycho-spiritual.

*Dementia in its worst case is obvious. The individual, who we consider to be our loved one, our parent, or our friend, is no longer there. We don't feel their personality. We don't feel their spirit. We just see somebody who is ... or a body that, communicates with us sometimes. At times they focus on us and sometimes they don't.*

*The longer they've been experiencing dementia, the more difficulty they're having in terms of understanding who we are and where we come from even if we're their children. This is the most difficult, including things like understanding or remembering things that happened thirty seconds or three or four minutes ago.*

*Those individuals who have experienced dementia in a limited sense—that being, in the short term, may apparently operate quite normally. Specifically, to those who they don't see very often. For instance, if you are living away from your parents' home and you still have two parents with one parent perfectly fine while the other has dementia. The parent who is perfectly fine will be saying that their partner is forgetful all the time, asks the same questions all the time, has difficulty in remembering things and is quite aggressive as a result. Then you as their child will come along once in a while, either you'll telephone them or you'll go and visit them, and they'll be perfectly clear of thought— they'll be totally focused. That's because you create a focus. As a temporary visitor you're not part of the "background" as is their partner, who is there all the time and therefore nonconsequential.*

*Everyday things and people who interact with the dementia patient don't create a focus for that individual, whereas when you as the child come along create a focus. As a result the person with dementia, the parent, starts to remember things straightaway, starts to understand who you are, what you are, what you are there for, and even down to conversations that you've had thirty to forty seconds ago.*

*However, the longer that you are there, you start to become part of the background again, and that's when things start to get repeated, and they start to forget things.*

*So, what is this focus? What is dementia, and what is it all about?*

*Well, it's really a way in which an aspect or soul has decided to leave the body. If you remember, there's a number of different termination junctures (ways to leave this incarnation) which we can have—up to five. The fifth one includes the final demise of the human form and the departure of the projected aspect from the True Energetic Self (sometimes called the Godhead or Oversoul or Higher Self, the aspect being called a soul, or an individualized unit of sentience and energy projected from the True Energetic Self). When it removes itself from that body, the vehicle that it is experiencing this particular environment with, demises.*

*With dementia, as an entity slowly moves out of the energies of the incarnate human vehicle, the association with it is gradually reduced, as is its ability to animate it. Ultimately the body dies.*

*It's a case of, "there is no longer a need to be incarnate." The soul is gradually moving out of the way. The expectations and the goals of the life plan have been, for all intents and purposes, completed, therefore some souls decide to go home. They either choose one of the departure or termination junctures or they finish their life plan close to the fifth termination juncture, and as a result their life plan is terminated at the same time.*

*However, although it may have satisfied the goals or the requirements of its life plan, it may have decided to stay a bit longer for those individuals it has become associated with in this particular incarnation, such as its partner or its family members.*

*Now we have a dichotomy, there's still a link with the human form, the incarnate human vehicle, but there's a desire from the incarnate aspect or soul to go back to the energetic and enter its previous level of communion with its True Energetic Self.*

*The aspect (soul) doesn't need to be here, doesn't really want to be here, but feels duty bound to be here for those who they feel are dependent upon them "being there" for confidence reasons, for emotional reasons, and basically for "maintaining that family unit" as well.*

*Dementia is, in a nutshell, the soul or the incarnate aspect gradually moving away from the incarnation, and rather than going rapidly, either through disease, illness, accident, or the longevity of the human vehicle just ending, its cognitive function breaks down until it is no longer functional.*

*To repeat myself, it's really about understanding that the aspect or soul is departing slowly and that the focus is awakened when we go and see them. For instance, if they're in a care facility and we go to see them, they suddenly wake up. This wake up is caused by a part of their sentience coming back to meet us. It comes back down the Hara Line—that little energetic tube that maintains the connectivity between the incarnate aspect and the True Energetic Self—and basically greets us, so to speak. From a human perspective, it doesn't feel that way, but from the soul or the aspects perspective, it would say: "Oh, I've got to be there for them" and they come back down the frequencies and the Hara Line. It's only when there's been a long period of "time," that the visitor starts to become part of the background and that they think: "Oh well, they know I'm here now, so I can start to drift back." And that's when we start to lose the essence of the individual and the lack of personality, lack of understanding, and the vacant look in the eyes of the individual with dementia starts to become prevalent again.*

*It is possible to see a link between dementia and being in a coma. This is because in the extreme cases of dementia, the body is just alive. From our human perspective, it's alive but it's not really animated or interactive in a correct way, in a way that is applicable to and associated with the full level of connectivity from an aspect. When we see people with dementia just sitting with a vacant look on their faces this is almost the same as being in a coma. Because in general comas can be contained or maintained by a very small percentage of sentience a lot of comas can be subsequently maintained by medical and mechanical means. Rather than having the eyes open with a vacant stare, because there's nobody there, there's very little sentience to animate the body, the eyes are generally closed.*

*Coma and dementia/Alzheimer's are almost identical in terms of what's going on; that being, the soul or incarnate aspect isn't in the body or isn't fully in the body.*

*When you see somebody with dementia, just recognize that they really aren't all there because the sentience and the energy that is associated with that body is mostly gone.*

*One can give them the opportunity to "go" if you want. You can give them the permission to go rather than perpetuating this condition, where they're sometimes here and sometimes not here, moving backward and forward to the body. Tell them that they can go now.*

*Moving back and forth, to and from the body is actually something that we do at the start of an incarnation, when we first associate ourselves with the human form in the fetus or in the embryonic state. We move back and forth when the body is first born or whether we're in a dementia state about to leave the body. We're backward and forward all the time. So really and truly, just accept or give these people permission to go. Just say to them: "You know, you don't need to hang around, you can go back to your True Energetic Self or you can go back Home." That will give them more incentive to go and detach the animating energy from the human form, removing it from the Tan Tien and the rest of the sentience from the Soul Seat and bringing it back toward the Core Star, moving it back up the Hara Line to return into communion with its True Energetic Self, allowing the body to demise accordingly.*

*If you see anybody with dementia, just recognize it's because their aspect or soul isn't fully integrated with the body, it's probably finished its life plan and is feeling no reason to be here other than to provide consolation or confidence or the need to "be there" for others who are part of the family unit.*

*That's what dementia is all about. It's about the aspect or soul leaving the body, but not quite removing the connection.*

# How We Incarnate, How It Affects Us Psychologically, and How to Heal Such Conditions, Including a Short Explanation for Bipolarism

One of the things that I have noticed over the years of healing is that some of the ways in which we incarnate can affect us in ways that cannot be explained by current psychological science. Indeed, it is difficult to state that psychology is a science. If it is, it's definitely not an exact one. That being said, the information referring to *how we incarnate and how it affects us* can also be classified as scientific if one considers that the way in which we incarnate, as a function, has a number of affects that can be both understood and healed. Some of course cannot be healed or treated because they are an operational condition and not a symptom or dysfunction.

In order to start with this section, I need to refer to some of the text that Anne, my late but still communicative energetic wife, partner, and OM soul mate, offered on the subject in *The Anne Dialogues*. First, we need to understand the structure associated with our True Energetic Self (TES). Where there is an ability to correct a psychological issue/s that is a function of the state of how we incarnate, I will illustrate the psycho-spiritual reprogramming available to the healer.

I will let Anne do the talking. Her communication is designated by the use of A: Before I do this, though, I would like to remind the readers that the TES is a unit of sentient energy that is individualized from the sentient energy that is The Source. This is or we are actually Source sentience given a body (group, volume, mass) of energy to enable it to experience the multiversal environment that is part of the overall structure of the Source. The Source, in turn, is a unit of sentience and energy individualized from The Origin. Sentience is what The Origin, The Source, and our TES "is." The energy is given, used, or appropriated by sentience to allow it to experience the environment it is in, in the way it is supposed to be experienced, as if it is part of that environment. Based upon this, our TES is actually a combination of our True Sentient Self (TSS), which is pure sentience and energy within which the sentience chooses to house itself.

## The Hierarchial Structure Associated with the TES

A: It's a delight to be able to work with you again. Although I will be going over the same ground as in our last dialogue, I will be changing some of the emphasis, specifically as I will be describing the way to find a healing solution to some of the ways in which we incarnate.

The True Energetic Self (TES) (*sometimes called the oversoul, higher self, or godhead —GSN*) can project up to twelve smaller Aspects of itself into any universal environment within the structure of the multiverse. These are what are sometimes described as Souls. I will, however, no longer use the word Soul, because it naturally associates the Aspect as being the "Self," the dominant sentience and not the TES as the True Self, the real dominate sentience. It is this error in thought that stops us as incarnate Aspects from moving outside of our understanding of self; that being, our association with the human vehicle being predominant in the physical universe.

There is a structure below the Aspect level, and this structure is where the Aspect itself can project up to twelve smaller Aspects of itself into other universal environments within the multiversal structure. These smaller Aspects are called Shards.

*(The TES can, in the most extreme case, have twelve Aspects projected with each Aspect projecting twelve Shards, making one hundred and forty-four individualizations of the TES. — GSN)*

A: Aspects and Shards experience individualization when projected from their TES or Aspect and so as with the Aspect in relationship to the TES, the Shard can and does experience true individuality while in the projected state. That being, it is capable of individual incarnations and the parallel conditions created by the Event Space associated with it.

The TES cannot commune with The Source until it has evolved through the structure of the multiverse and all of its projected Aspects are back in a state of communion with it. This is similar with the projected Aspect in relation to its Shards. The projected Aspect cannot commune with its TES until all of its Shards are reintegrated with it. Note the use of the word reintegration relative to the Shard rather than communion. This is because the Shard, being of significantly reduced sentience in comparison to the Aspect, cannot enter into any of the states of communion in the individualized state I previously described.

*(A Shard is only individualized while in the projected state, and it is always reintegrated with the Aspect when its role, incarnate or other, is finished. —GSN)*

A: An incarnating Shard is not usually capable of thinking of itself as being anything other than the vehicle it incarnates into, such is the level of sentience associated with it.

A Shard can be an individual projection or a partial (single) migration of sentience. The rule surrounding the percentage of overall sentience that can be projected from an Aspect to create its Shards is the same as for a TES projecting its sentience to create its Aspects. This is that there is always 70 percent of the sentience that remains in the main body of the TES, and therefore there is always 70 percent of the sentience that remains in the main body of the Aspect.

The sentience associated with an Aspect projected from its TES is circa 2 1/2 percent of the total sentience of the TES and the sentient functionality associated with it. This is the same for the percentage of sentience that a Shard is allowed to have in general from its Aspect, which would create a limitation in the ability to think outside of the incarnate self.

The Shard that is a single migration of sentience into another incarnate vehicle can, if the Aspect has no other Shards projected, assign the full 30 percent of its available sentience for projection to that Shard. This is the same for an Aspect if the TES was only using a single migration of sentience into another incarnate vehicle. This means that in the case of the TES, it would have its own experiences at the same time as the Aspect its sentience was migrated into.

The TES experiences the ability to drive its own energies and the incarnate vehicle its migrated sentience is in at the same time which is normal for the TES because that is how it experiences things via its projections generally. With the exception, that is, that the projected Aspects drive the incarnate vehicle they are projected into, whereas in this instance, the TES is driving the incarnate vehicle on behalf of its migrated sentience. Think of it in terms of driving two motor cars at the same time.

This is the same for the Aspect that migrates its sentience into a Shard but with a slight difference because the TES that migrates its sentience is not incarnate but the Aspect that projects its sentience is. In this instance, the Aspect being already incarnate is usually incarnate at a frequency within the physical universe where it retains a large proportion of its connectivity with its TES. It also enjoys the functionality associated with that frequency which includes the command and control of the energies associated with its environment, which includes the incarnate vehicle it occupies.

A Shard cannot think of itself as an independent entity. However, if the Shard was projected and was given autonomy it would do, and the Aspect would receive the experiences in the normal parallel way a TES with a projected Aspect and an Aspect with a projected Shard are recorded. But because the sentience and its associated energies are in the state of migration, the Aspect drives both the incarnate vehicle it resides within and the incarnate vehicle its Shard is incarnate into. In this instance, the sentience in its state of migration is split between the two vehicles and drives both of them, it drives both motor cars if you like, at the same time and experiences everything in both vehicles concurrently as a single function of sentience. In summary, the Shard does not think of itself as a single autonomic entity; it is simply an extension of the Aspect's sentience, and thinks of itself as being both the Shard and Aspect, just as the Aspect thinks of itself as the Shard as well. It's just that the sentience is in two vehicles.

## Maintained Connectivity with Event Space

*Anne continues ...*

A: An incarnate Aspect that has maintained connectivity with Event Space is one that can either traverse all of the potential realities associated with its dualistic, trilistic, or quadrulistic decisions, etc., at will, or is forever confused as to where it is and what it has achieved.

In respect of the incarnate Aspect that is in control of this function, it can achieve two things. First, it can position itself into the alternative events that may, could, or will present themselves to it and make an active decision as to which decision is optimal or desirable. Or second, it can communicate with those versions of itself that exist within these alternative realities and accelerate its own experiential and evolutionary content in the process.

This is relative to any of the versions of the incarnate Aspect that are created as a result of the creation of additional Event Spaces due to the decisions that the primary incarnate Aspect has made, and/or the decision of the other fractalized versions. Each of them will consider that they are the primary incarnate Aspect existing in the primary Event Space. Normally none of them will recognize that they are the product of a previous decision and are therefore another version, a copy, so to speak. The only exception to this condition is the Aspect that incarnates with the ability to experience these different Event Spaces, these different realities, at will, knowing that it could be either the primary incarnation or one of the copies while not being affected by this thought process.

Incarnate Aspects have been doing this for some time and are called psychics. Most of them, though, are not able to use this function to its true potential. If it is aware and awake it will be in acceptance of the ultimate possibilities just discussed, and it will also be able to use the ability to project its consciousness into the Event Spaces occupied by those other versions of itself that it is experiencing. In essence, the Aspect that has the capability of experiencing the Event Spaces (while controlling its own Event Space) of other versions of itself will benefit (as will its primary Aspect and TES) from its ability to experience parallel existences by accruing the evolutionary content associated with these experiences and the evolutionary content associated with the ability to experience them concurrently rather than linearly.

Those incarnate Aspects that have either the ability to see or experience the myriad downstream Event Spaces associated with its own downstream potential Event Space/s in an uncontrollable way—that being, they don't have the awareness that is normally associated with such functionality—have a very hard time anchoring themselves to their current Event Space. They will experience things that their friends, relatives, and associates will not be able to relate to because some Event Spaces will be in the far future, or variations of a far future from a chronological perspective that could or may be diversified from its main line Event Space and the fractalizations from it. They will be considered psychotic and unless they can be educated as to what is happening to them, including being trained to control this function, they run a great risk of being institutionalized.

Similarly, those incarnate Aspects that have ability to project their consciousness into the incarnate Aspects associated with the other versions of themselves in an uncontrollable way, including their downstream potential Event Spaces, will also have significant difficulty in working in their current Event Space. Their consciousness will move seamlessly from one Event Space to another, experiencing them as if they are one Event Space but without the continuity associated with being in the same line of Event Space. Any continuity errors experienced will create profound psychological issues because roles and tasks that they have undertaken may not be relevant in their Event Space or the roles and tasks that they should have done in their Event Space may not be actioned as a result of these errors. They will also have difficulty interfacing with people in their career, relationships, and recreational pastimes. They will not know what their reality is, how valid it is, and whether their memories/actions are real or fiction. Again, without the correct level of education and training they will be considered psychotic and run a great risk of being institutionalized.

## Walk-Ins

There are four main types of Walk-Ins and incarnate mankind experiences them as:

1. One-to-one Walk-Ins
2. Multiple Walk-Ins
3. Multiple non-animate or passive Walk-Ins
4. Single temporary/permanent, active or passive Walk-Ins

*A possible fifth is when a walk-in wants to take over control of the incarnate human form from the primary Aspect which is not part of the original life plan.*

*Again, Anne continues ...*

## One-to-One Walk-Ins

A: One-to-one Walk-Ins are what spiritualists generally recognize as a Walk-In. This is best described in two ways. First, it can be the result of an Aspect deciding that it has learned, experienced, and evolved enough from a particular incarnation, wants to return to the energetic, and subsequently desires the incarnate vehicle to be used by another Aspect because there is enough longevity in the vehicle to make a Walk-In viable. Or second, it made a decision prior to initiation, prior to integrating itself into the incarnate process, that as part of its life plan it would leave the physical state at a predetermined point and another known Aspect would take over the incarnate vehicle and continue the incarnation in accordance with its own life plan and that created by the first Aspect to incarnate into the incarnate vehicle. In this instance, the primary incarnating Aspect can choose to experience any length of incarnate experience from a few seconds to the whole incarnation with all but a few seconds. The secondary incarnating Aspect therefore can Walk-In to experience incarnate existence from the perspective of almost a whole incarnation, if the primary Aspect only desired to experience the conception, gestation period, and birth of the fetus, to the final few moments of the incarnation in the incarnate vehicle, which would include the demise process.

The psychological aspects of a Walk-In are loss of memory (of varying levels and durations), changes in personality, disorientation, and reduction of, or increase in, skill set/s.

*As this is a simple function of the change of one Aspect for another Aspect in the same incarnate vehicle there are considered to be no adverse psychological affects and so no psycho-spiritual healing is necessary. Possible healing would be the education of the family members and friends surrounding the incarnate human vehicle of the reasons for personality changes etc. —GSN*

## Multiple Walk-Ins

A: Are a condition where the incarnate vehicle is used by either a known or an indeterminate number of Aspects throughout the longevity of the incarnate vehicle. In terms of the known number of Aspects using the incarnate vehicle, each of the Aspects that associated themselves with the vehicle as part of their life plan will have decided which or what part of the "life" they will be incarnate within the vehicle for, the total number of incarnations creating a whole coherent life from the perspective of the external incarnate Aspect that is in the "immersed" state of incarnation and is therefore not aware and awake to the point of recognizing the incarnate vehicle it sees as being anything other than one person, one body.

From the psychological aspect the only issue here is that a long-term associate (friend) would see a gradual change in the personality of their friend over the years they know them, the changes being specific to when the Walk-Ins swap out.

In terms of the incarnate vehicle being used by an indeterminate number of Aspects, there is almost no plan to the "life" the incarnated vehicle will have. This is because those Aspects that use the vehicle will incarnate when and where the opportunity arises—that being when the currently incumbent Aspect decides that it has experienced enough, or its "life plan" has been satisfied. They will of course have their own life plan but it will not correlate or link in to the overall life experienced by the incarnate vehicle, their plan being able to experience what they can, when they can, and doing their best to work with the conditions of the life and its environment that it inherits from the previous Aspect.

From the psychological aspect the external observer would see a completely irrational change in behavior and personality of the incarnate vehicle over its longevity due to the lack of planning in integration with the experiences and environment the incarnate vehicle is exposed to with previously coherent or incoherent decision-making processes being negated and replaced with those associated with the newly incarnating Aspect. The external observer may also note additional specialisms being displayed by the incarnate vehicle that are specific to the Aspects that walk in.

*No psycho-spiritual healing is necessary unless the irrational changes observed are mentally or physically violent toward others. Further healing would be the education of the family members and friends surrounding the incarnate human vehicle of the reasons for personality changes, etc. See "Multiple or Single, Temporary or Permanent, Active or Passive Walk-Ins That Want to Keep or Take Control." —GSN*

## Multiple nonanimate (passive) temporary Walk-Ins

A: Are totally unrelated to multiple Walk-Ins. These Walk-Ins are a function of the desire of a number of Aspects to experience the incarnate existence of the primary incarnate Aspect on a temporary basis while being in the passive role. That being, they are not in control of the animation of the incarnate vehicle. Provided the primary incarnate Aspect is in accordance with the addition or subtraction of multiple passive Walk-Ins, the number of different Aspects can change or swap out almost on a daily basis.

There is no obvious psychological function of this Walk-In that can be observed by the external observer because the incarnate vehicle is animated by the primary Aspect only, with no interference to the life plan from the passive Walk-Ins.

*No psycho-spiritual healing is necessary. — GSN*

## Multiple nonanimate (passive) permanent Walk-Ins

A: Are a function of the desire of a number of Aspects to experience the incarnate existence of the primary incarnate Aspect while being in the passive role throughout the total longevity of the incarnate vehicle. As with the Walk-In condition just mentioned they are not in control of the animation of the incarnate vehicle, they are simply back-seat passengers, so to speak.

As with the previous condition there is no obvious psychological function of this Walk-In that can be observed by the external observer because the incarnate vehicle is animated by the primary Aspect only. In both this instance and the previous instance of the multiple Walk-In, the only way the presence of the other Aspects would be noted would be in regressive or "in-depth" hypnosis.

*No psycho-spiritual healing is necessary. — GSN*

## Single temporary active Walk-Ins

A: Are Walk-Ins that occupy the incarnate vehicle at the same time as the primary incarnate Aspect and have the ability to animate (control) the incarnate vehicle. Animation is either achieved in isolation to, in parallel with, or in tandem with the primary incarnate Aspect.

From the psychological perspective, the

outside observer would witness similar behavior patterns to those presented by the incarnate vehicle that experiences multiple Walk-Ins.

*No psycho-spiritual healing is necessary. — GSN*

### Single temporary passive Walk-Ins

A: Are Walk-Ins that occupy the incarnate vehicle at the same time as the primary incarnate Aspect on a temporary basis, but which don't have the ability to animate (control) the incarnate vehicle. In this instance, the temporary passive Walk-In is, as with the multiple passive Walk-In, a purely back-seat passenger, observing and experiencing the existence and life plan of the primary incarnate Aspect but not influencing it.

From the psychological perspective, the outside observer would not witness any unfamiliar behavior patterns to those presented by the primary incarnate vehicle. The only way to identify that the incarnate vehicle housed a temporary Aspect would be via regressive hypnosis.

*No psycho-spiritual healing is necessary. — GSN*

### Single permanent passive Walk-Ins

A: Are Walk-Ins that occupy the incarnate vehicle at the same time as the primary incarnate Aspect on a permanent basis, but which don't have the ability to animate (control) the incarnate vehicle. In this instance, the permanent passive Walk-In is, as with the multiple permanent Walk-In, a purely back-seat passenger, observing and experiencing the existence and life plan of the primary incarnate Aspect but not influencing it.

From the psychological perspective, the outside observer would not witness any unfamiliar behavior patterns to those presented by the primary incarnate vehicle. The only way to identify that the incarnate vehicle housed a temporary Aspect would be via regressive hypnosis.

*No psycho-spiritual healing is necessary. — GSN*

## Walk-Ins That Want to Keep or Take Control

*I was about to say something about the content in this section of the final chapter of this book of illustrations of healing techniques or modalities, when that other Aspect of my OM TES, Anne (the sentient energy, that is), decided that it would like to make further comments before describing how to deal with such issues.*

A: Although I have described most of the information that you have taken from *The Anne Dialogues* to show deeper levels of "Walk-In," I want to give your readers an illustration of the reason why a Walk-In would want to take control of the incarnate human vehicle they are associated with. This association can of course be with multiple or single, temporary or permanent, active or passive Walk-Ins that want to keep or take control.

ME: OK, please explain why an Aspect would wish to do such a thing.

A: In essence Walk-Ins are allowed to "Walk-In" because of a number of reasons. They are:

1. That they only need to experience one thing within the incarnation of a specific Aspect and that this does not justify the use of a whole incarnation within which the benefits to another Aspect may be greater.
2. There is an agreement with the TES of the incarnate Aspect that occupied the incarnate human vehicle first, that when the life plan is complete, the incarnate human vehicle can be

vacated and used by another Aspect. This is in exception to the incarnate Aspect taking on additional evolutionary opportunity/ies.

3. There is a need (can be a preplanned need) for the experience of another Aspect to assist the primary incarnate Aspect in some way.
4. The availability of incarnate human vehicle, or other incarnate vehicles within the physical universe and its frequencies, is limited versus demand and so Aspects can share an incarnate human, or other vehicle, sharing the control of the interaction with other incarnates. It is not uncommon for four or more Aspects to be passively attached to an incarnate human vehicle with just one being active and therefore controlling or being the primary animation force for the incarnate human vehicle. Although not strictly a Walk-In it can be dealt with in the same way as described later on in this section.
5. That the incarnate human vehicle is in a position of leadership and needs the experience and evolutionary content of more than one Aspect.
6. The primary incarnate Aspect has a desire to terminate its incarnation but does not want to commit suicide or waste the longevity of the incarnate human vehicle it is currently incumbent within. Another suitable Aspect is then authorized to "swap out" with the primary incarnate Aspect.
7. One or more Aspects are allowed to be "passive" passengers so to speak either for the total duration of the incarnation of the primary incarnate Aspect or for parts of its incarnation.
8. One or more of the active or passive Aspects have decided that they can do a better job than

the primary incarnate Aspect.

A: There are other Walk-Ins, though, that are not so benevolent.

ME: Go on.

A: Those Walk-Ins that happen when

1. The primary Aspect has abused the incarnate human vehicle by the use of substance abuse (drugs) or alcohol, in which case the incarnate human vehicle's frequencies becomes so low that the incarnate Aspect is either temporally ejected out of, or removes itself temporarily, from the incarnate human body until the effect of the substance or alcohol is reduced and its frequencies are returned to an acceptable condition for the Aspect to return. In this instance, Aspects that are "Earth bound" i.e. those that are still seeking an incarnate existence because they refuse to move on back up the frequencies and communion with their TES want to experience incarnation, no matter how short it is. In this instance, they accept the disharmony associated with the incarnate vehicle not being frequentially or energetically aligned to them either naturally or due to the abuse. Simply put, they suffer pain to incarnate temporarily. Due to the level of disharmony experienced the Walk-In usually displays an angry and violent demeanor—again an obvious change in personality. The Walk-In can only walk-in while the primary or normally incumbent Aspect is absent. There is a natural ejection process that happens when the primary Aspect is able to return. This usually results in a peak of anger and a sudden loss of consciousness (the paralytic response)

followed by the return of the primary Aspect and the normal personality. Loss of memory is normal as is a headache.

2. Aspects are addicted to the sensations associated with incarnation and seek to take control of the incarnate human vehicle when they can, such as when the incarnate human vehicle energies are low during illness or during sleep. They can attach themselves to a certain incarnate human vehicle and its Aspect and feel its feelings of attraction to certain sensations or addictive behaviors.
3. Astral entities can try to experience incarnation with any of the above two aggressive Walk-In examples. You have already dealt with the removal of astral entities/beings but they can also be considered as removable in the same way and process described in the last section.

There are two healing modalities that can be used to correct all of the above conditions

1. Compartmentalize the Aspect/s that are authorized as passive or active Walk-Ins but that are trying to or have taken over control of the incarnate human vehicle.
2. Eject or remove those Aspects that have Walked-In to the incarnate human vehicle in a time of energetic weakness being experienced by the primary incarnate Aspect.

A: You have of course experience of both of these healing modalities so I will let you continue with your description. I may decide to "chip in" if I think it's relevant.

Don't forget. The most obvious evidence of a Walk-In is a change in personality, traits, and/or habits.

ME: Thank you for your help. It was very useful.

A: It's my pleasure. I look forward to our next venture!

## Compartmentalizing or Reassignation of Control

The comment from Anne about the change (sometimes sudden) in personality, traits, or habits of someone you know is a very robust way of identifying if an incarnate human vehicle has experienced a Walk-In or a bid to take over control of the body. More often than not it is obvious and as a result the friends and loved ones should be tolerant and seek a psycho-spiritual solution rather than a physical or medical one. Addiction, of course, sometimes needs physical assistance as well as psycho-spiritual help.

Bipolarism is usually a function of two Aspects associated with the incarnate human vehicle alternating for command and control of the human vehicle.

Once assistance has been sought from the healer and authority to be healed gained, the healer can work on the patient that displays the elements of a Walk-In or passive Aspect that has taken over control from the primary incarnate "animating" Aspect.

I very often see multiple Aspects arguing over command and control of an incarnate human vehicle looking like a number of spoilt children in a car or in a series of rooms in a house. One of the rooms is the control room, which allows an Aspect the capability of animating or controlling the incarnate human vehicle that they are associated to albeit in a supposedly passive nature. In the car illustration, it's like they are fighting to be in the driver seat!!

The only way to affect a healing and allow the primary incarnate Aspect to regain control of the human vehicle they are assigned to is to reestablish control by compartmentalization.

In order to do this, raise your frequencies by opening your chakras to the seventh level and use your intention to elevate yourself to the eleventh frequency. Again, you are outside of the frequencies associated with the incarnate human vehicle, which is necessary in this process.

Visualize yourself having an aerial view of the incarnate human vehicle and the Aspects that are associated with it. See them in a control room with other rooms next to it where the control room is normally closed or off limits to other inhabitants, with the other inhabitants in the other rooms but able to see what's going on in the control room through a glass wall or TV screen. In the context of the car, consider it like a taxi or limousine where the driver normally has a protective shield or glass between them and the passengers.

Whichever visualization you use the general process is the same. In this instance, therefore, I will use the image of the control room and adjoining rooms as observed from above, the aerial view I just mentioned. I will also use a total of four Aspects to illustrate the process. One being the primary incarnate.

Visualize each of the Aspects within the building in a room of their own, each room is arranged so that they have a view of the control room where the primary incarnate Aspect can control the incarnate human vehicle. The control room is an equilateral triangle and the adjoining rooms are square with one wall adjoining one side of the triangular control room. Each has a clear glass wall where they adjoin the triangular room so that they can see what is happening. Now look and see that these walls are not solid, each of them has a doorway through their glass wall and into the control room and that there are four Aspects in the control room and not one (they may look like human beings but could of course be in energetic "orb"-based form!). Note that they are quarreling or fighting to take a turn at being at the control room and therefore being the primary Aspect in control of the incarnate human vehicle.

## Conceptual Image of the Triangular Control Room and the Three Rooms the Passive Aspects Should Be In

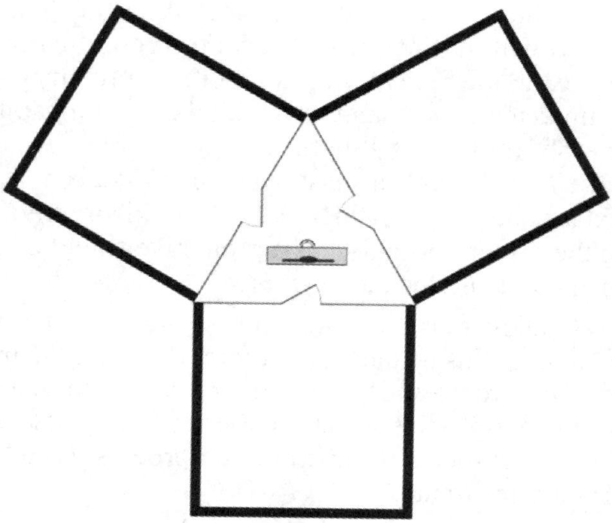

With four Aspects fighting over the control of the incarnate human vehicle, it is no wonder that people who are immersed in their incarnation think that the person who is recognized as their friend, colleague, or partner is having a psychotic issue. The primary Aspect will be obvious to see. It will be a golden color, whereas the others will be darker. This golden color represents a higher level of natural integration with the incarnate human vehicle, that of the primary Aspect.

Use your energetic hand to move one of the Aspects that should be in a passive and observational state back into one of the rooms. It doesn't matter which one. Gently "herd" the Aspect into the room. Be careful, it will be resourceful and try to move around your hand and make its way back into the control room. You may even see the other Aspects try to help it (not the primary Aspect, though). Once you have herded it into one of the rooms with your energetic hand, close the door. Because you are operating at a higher frequency you will be able to pass through the door without issue or problem, the Aspect you herded will not. Move outside of the door and visualize three strong locks (and three appropriate keys in your hand) on the long edge of the door. Lock each lock one by one. Once the door is fully locked the door will disappear and the wall will become a single wall of glass.

You have now isolated one of the Aspects that was trying to become active when it was supposed to be passive.

Follow the same process and procedure with the other two Aspects one by one. Note that they will be more evasive now because one of them has been returned back to the passive state. But to reiterate:

Use your energetic hand to move the second Aspect that should be in a passive and observational state back into one of the rooms. It doesn't matter which one of the two that is left. Gently "herd" the Aspect into the room. Be careful; it will be resourceful and try to move around your hand and make its way back into the control room. It will have learned from the first Aspect to be compartmentalized what is going to happen to it. You may even see the other Aspect try to help it. Once you have herded it into one of the remaining two rooms with your energetic hand, close the door. Move outside of the door and visualize the three strong locks and the appropriate keys in your hand. Lock each lock one by one. Once the door is fully locked, it will disappear in the same way as the first and the wall will become a single wall of glass.

You have now isolated one of the second Aspects that was trying to become active when it was supposed to be passive.

Repeat the process for the third and final Aspect and the third and final square room.

Now all you have left is the primary Aspect in the triangular room. The doors to the other rooms are now dissolved with the now passive Aspects behind their observational glass windows. To finalize the work, use your intention to use the control panel in the primary

Aspect's triangular room to program the windows to the three square rooms to be one-way glass, where the primary Aspect cannot see the passive Aspects but the passive Aspects can see the primary Aspect and its work. That being the primary Aspect cannot see the other passive Aspects and so they cannot influence it in any way. This simple but effective visualization returns the primary Aspect into full control of the incarnate human vehicle, as it should be.

Finish by descending the frequencies by using your intention to move from the eleventh frequency to the seventh and then close each chakra until you are back on the Earth or zero level. Both you and the patient should drink some water to help ground yourselves.

## Removal of a Walk-In

There are times when the healer needs to actually remove a Walk-In from the incarnate human vehicle. More often than not this is because its presence is either not planned or planned and no longer required with the Aspect that is no longer required wanting to stay in the state of being a Walk-In.

In both of these instances and those commented upon by Anne above, the Walk-In needs to be removed by the healer. The primary reason for the Walk-In to be removed in these instances is because it affects the proper and correct function of the primary incarnate Aspect in an adversarial or detrimental way.

Removing a Walk-In is actually quite an easy process and as a result is very effective in terms of healing the psychological issues that are displayed by the patient.

In order to remove a Walk-In the healer needs to raise their own frequencies to at least the eleventh frequency level using the process that is by now well known to the reader.

Once at the eleventh level, visualize the control room described in the previous section. Within the control room will be both the primary incarnate Aspect and the Walk-In. Again, they may appear to be in human form but could of course be in energetic "orb"-based form. Irrespective of the form that they take use your intention to create a doorway in the control room. You can make it the same triangular shape as the control room in the last section if you wish. Now create a smaller, temporary room that is only accessible from the control room; this will be used to compartmentalize the Walk-In, that is to be removed. Use your energetic hand to herd the unwanted Aspect into the smaller, temporary room. Note that it may create some form of resistance. Ignore the resistance and gently herd or move the Walk-In into the room. Once the Walk-In is in the temporary room, use your intention to dissolve the doorway into the room. Now detach the room from the main control room that the primary Aspect uses to command and control (animate) the incarnate human vehicle that it is associated to.

The temporary room is now separated from the control room of the incarnate human vehicle and can be used as a vehicle in its own right to transport the Walk-In, to allow it to be returned to its TES. Focus on the TES of the Walk-In; meditate on sending it a message stating that you have one of its Aspects and that it needs to reenter into communion with it. Concentrate on the TES of the Walk-In, feel its presence, feel it close to you. When you feel and "know" that it is close to you, use your energetic hand/s to give the room with its Walk-In Aspect within it to it, hand it back to it in the same way that you might return a lost item to its owner. Visualize this happening, see the TES energetically take hold of the room with the Walk-In Aspect within it and absorb it within its own energies. The Walk-In has now returned to its TES of origin and the patient is no longer affected by the distractive influences of the unwanted Walk-in and its normal personality traits will return.

Finish by descending the frequencies by using your intention to move from the eleventh frequency to the seventh and then close each chakra until you are back on the Earth or zero level. Both you and the patient should drink some water to help ground yourselves.

## Psycho-Spiritual Method of Healing Uncontrolled Event Space Interaction

The best way to heal a client that is illustrating uncontrolled and random movement of their consciousness from one Event Space to another is to sever the links between the patient and those other Aspects of itself that they are interacting with.

In one instance of this I have experienced my client was moving in a totally random and uncontrolled way between this Event Space and what I perceived to be two other versions of themselves in two other Event Spaces. The person concerned was exhibiting anxiety, depression, worry, and a total lack of confidence. Indeed, the client was regularly showing frustration and was angry toward their family, especially when they "knew" that they had done something that they needed to do but that work was not in this Event Space (but was done in another!). Even more frustrating was when the client was told and even congratulated on the quality of work that they had done but that they had no memory of doing. The client came to my attention when a family member asked for help. The client was about to be put on medication when the family member contacted me for help. They were all at the end of their tether and understandably so.

The healing process I will describe is the one I used in the above example. Assuming that the reader is now fully conversant with the method I have described to elevate the frequencies of the healer by the use of the chakras, that is by opening them, I will not describe the process but will simply refer to it as a necessary process.

This healing can be performed either remotely or with the client or patient in the therapy room of the healer.

In all instances gain permission from the client or patient to perform it. Permission can be gained either verbally or energetically. If energetically is the only option please be aware of any egotistical desires to gain permission. If you don't get permission you cannot and will not be able to help the patient or client.

Either with the client or patient in your therapy room, or if you are performing a remote healing, sit in a straight-backed chair with your back straight/erect, place your hands palms upper most on your upper thighs, where the legs meet the lower body. Close your eyes and focus gently on the origin of the spiritual or third eye. Open all of your chakras one by one until you have reached the seventh chakra and therefore the seventh frequency level. Now use your intention to move up the last three frequencies associated with the incarnate human vehicle, the eighth, ninth, and tenth. Finally use your intention to move your consciousness to the eleventh frequency. This takes you outside the frequencies associated with the incarnate human vehicle and enables you to see the Hara Line connected to the step-down frequencies of the eighth, ninth, and tenth and the energetic templates that start at the seventh frequency level.

If you focus your intention correctly (use the visual capabilities of your spiritual or third eye), you will also be able to see the Hara Line disappearing up the frequencies to the location of the TES.

Now look for another energy line, one that is going away from the patient and disappearing into nothingness but with that nothingness being surrounded by a very thin and totally transparent outside line of a spherical bubble. This outside line of the bubble represents the demarcation between this Event Space, the one that you and the patient are focused upon working within, and the Event Space that another Aspect of the patient is working within. The energy line going to that spherical bubble is the connection between the patient in this Event Space and the other Aspect of the patient in the other Event Space.

Look again with more focus and you may well see other energy lines doing the same thing. Connecting the patient in this Event Space and the other Aspects of the patient in other Event Spaces. In the example above there were two others so let's assume this to be the same. In this respect, you would see two energy lines, normally attached via the heart chakras (front and back aspects). The front aspect of the heart chakra is the connection to one version of the patient in the first Event Space the other via the rear aspect of the heart chakra to the second Event Space. The connectivity between the patient's heart chakras in the other Event Spaces are normally observed to be in "series" similar to that of a battery terminal; that is, positive to negative to positive, etc. In this instance, it is seen as the front heart chakra of the patient in this "normal" Event Space connected to the rear aspect of heart chakra of the other Aspect of the patient in the first Event Space with the front heart chakra of that Aspect of the patient connected to the rear aspect of heart chakra in the other Aspect of the patient in the second Event Space, with the front aspect of the heart chakra in the Aspect of the patient in the second Event Space being connected to the rear aspect of the patient in this "normal "Event Space." *(This is a very long but necessary sentence I note. Apologies! —GSN)*

## Illustration of an Aspect Being Connected to Itself Represented in Other Event Spaces

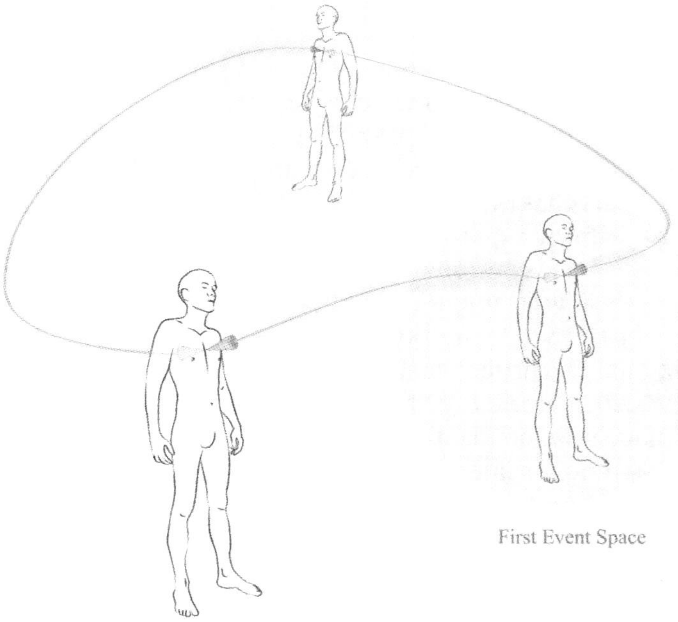


In this way, the patient is connected in a very robust and complete way with the three (in this example, three includes this current and "normal" Event Space) versions of themselves that their sentience is uncontrollably moving from and to.

Note these two things. First, it is not uncommon for the energy lines to be attached to other chakras or to be simply attached to one of the energy templates of the patient. Removal will be the same process even though the location of attachment is different. Second, if only one other Event Space is observed by the healer then the patient will normally be connected in the front to rear chakra aspect described above. The normal location is via the heart chakra simply because it is the closest chakra to the Soul Seat, the location of the sentience of the incarnate Aspect within the incarnate human vehicle.

Visualize yourself disconnecting the energy link from the front aspect of the heart chakra of your patient. Think of the electric lead with its plug and socket example previously used in the chapter on removing energy links between people. You can also use the simpler "hook and cable" illustrations in that chapter if it's easier for you. Disconnect the lead and plug from the socket in the center vortex (as a combination or assembly) of the front aspect of the heart chakra of your patient. Now remove the socket from the front aspect of the heart chakra by using your energetic hands to remove the center vortex of the heart chakra. Use your intention to create your recycling bin by the right-hand side of you and that you have a shelf full of spare chakra vortices just above the recycling bin. Select a new center vortex for the front aspect of a heart chakra and place it in the location of the vortex that you removed. You have now sealed off any potential for the rear aspect of the patients Aspect in the first Event Space to reconnect with the front aspect of the heart chakra of the patient in this event Space.

Now follow the disconnected energy line that is connected to the rear aspect of the heart chakra in the Aspect of the patient that is in the first Event Space. Use your intention to move inside the spherical bubble that represents the demarcation line of the first Event Space with your normal Event Space. Notice how you feel when you pass through it. Energetically you may find that it has a different feel about it. You may feel that you shouldn't be there! The bubble of Event Space demarcation will self-seal behind you. You are now in the first Event Space! Now disconnect the energy line and its connector (electric lead and plug in this example) from the connector (socket in this example) in the central vortex of the rear aspect of the heart chakra of the Aspect of the patient in this first Event Space. Discard both the energy line and the central vortex/socket assembly into your recycling bin, which will always be where you visualized it in the first instance, at your right-hand side—irrespective of which

Event Space you are in. In a similar way, you will see the shelf above the recycling bin with spare chakra vortices on the shelf. Replace the central vortex of the rear aspect of the heart chakra of the Aspect of your patient that is in this first Event Space.

You have now isolated the possibility of the connection between the front aspect of the heart chakra and your patient in your normal Event Space and the rear aspect of the heart chakra of your patient in the first Event Space.

However, there is still a connection between your patient in your normal Event Space and the Aspect of your patient in the first Event Space. This is via the connections between your patient in your normal Event Space via the rear aspect of the heart chakra of your patient in their normal Event Space and the front aspect or the heart chakra in the Aspect of your patient in the second Event Space. This is together with its connection to the Aspect of your patient in the first Event Space via the connection between the rear aspect of the heart chakra of the Aspect of your patient in the second Event Space and the front aspect of the heart chakra of the Aspect of your patient in the first Event Space.

Convoluted, isn't it!!!

Getting on with it then!

Move to the front aspect of the heart chakra of the Aspect of your patient in the first Event Space. Remove the energy link from the front aspect of the heart chakra of your patient in this first Event Space. Again, use the visualization of the electric lead with its plug and socket example. Disconnect the lead and plug from the socket that will be in the center vortex of the front aspect of the heart chakra of your patient in this first Event Space. Now remove the socket from the front aspect of the heart chakra by using your energetic hands to remove the center vortex of the heart chakra. Discard the socket and central vortices assembly into your recycling bin. From the shelf full of spare chakra vortices just above the recycling bin select a new center vortex for the front aspect of a heart chakra in this first Event Space and place it in the location of the vortex that you removed. You have now sealed off any potential for the rear aspect of the patients Aspect in the second Event Space to reconnect with the front aspect of the heart chakra of the patient in the first Event Space.

Now follow the disconnected energy line that is connected to the rear aspect of the heart chakra in the Aspect of the patient that is in the second Event Space. Use your intention to move inside the spherical bubble that represents the demarcation line of the second Event Space with the first Event Space (and even your Event Space!). Notice again how you feel when you pass through into it. Energetically you may find that it has an even different feel about it. You may experience a greater feeling that you shouldn't be there! The bubble of Event Space demarcation will self-seal behind you as you pass from the first Event Space into the second Event Space. You are now in the second Event Space! Now disconnect the energy line and its connector (electric lead and plug in this example) from the connector (socket in this example) in the central vortex of the rear aspect of the heart chakra of the Aspect of the patient in this Second Event Space. Discard both the energy line and the central vortex/socket assembly into your recycling bin. From the spare chakra vortices on the shelf replace the central vortex of the rear aspect of the heart chakra of the Aspect of your patient that is in this second Event Space.

Only now have you totally isolated the connectivity between your patient in their normal Event Space and the Aspect of your patient in the first Event Space.

Move to the front aspect of the heart chakra of the Aspect of your patient in the second Event Space.

Remove the energy link from the front aspect of the heart chakra of your patient in this second Event Space. Again, use the visualization of the electric lead with its plug and socket example. Disconnect the lead and plug from the socket that will be in the center vortex of the front aspect of the heart chakra of your patient in this second Event Space. Now remove the socket from the front aspect of the heart chakra by using your energetic hands to remove the center vortex of the heart chakra. Discard the socket and central vortices assembly into your recycling bin. From the shelf full of spare chakra vortices just above the recycling bin select a new center vortex for the front aspect of a heart chakra in this second Event Space and place it in the location of the vortex that you removed. You have now sealed off any potential for the rear aspect of the patient's Aspect in the normal Event Space to reconnect with the front aspect of the heart chakra of the patient in the second Event Space.

One more piece of work to do to complete the disconnection.

Now follow the disconnected energy line that is connected to the rear aspect of the heart chakra in the Aspect of the patient that is in the normal Event Space. Use your intention to move inside the spherical bubble that represents the demarcation line of the normal Event Space with the second Event Space (and even the first Event Space!). Notice again how you feel when you pass through into it. It will feel normal! The bubble of Event Space demarcation will self-seal behind you as you pass from the second Event Space into the normal Event Space. You are now back in your normal Event Space! Now disconnect the energy line and its connector in the central vortex of the rear aspect of the heart chakra of the Aspect of the patient in this normal Event Space. Discard both the energy line and the central vortex/socket assembly into your recycling bin. From the spare chakra vortices on the shelf replace the central vortex of the rear aspect of the heart chakra of the Aspect of your patient that is in this normal Event Space.

Now that you have completed the disconnection of your patient from the other two Event Spaces you can descend down the frequencies by using your intention to move from the eleventh frequency to the seventh and then closing the chakras until you are at the Earth or zero level. Both you and your patient are advised to take a drink of water to help ground you.

You have now totally disconnected the connectivity between the three aspects of your patient in the three separate Event Spaces. This includes the random and uncontrollable switching or experience of your patient's sentience with these Event Spaces.

In my experience this process is only one of a number of ways in which a patient displaying the random and uncontrollable projection of their sentience from one Event Space to another can be healed. Although I have a couple of other ways of performing this modality of psycho-spiritual healing, this one is the easiest and actually the most robust, even if it is long winded!

# Afterword

This book on my healing modalities is not a definitive list of what is available to the patient by me or any other healer. This is because energetic/vibrational healing and psycho-spiritual healing is an expansive subject that is as diverse as the patients that need healing.

The basics are here to be absorbed and considered by the experienced healer. I do not suggest the use of this book as a training handbook. It is simply a guide, a window, as to what is available and possible should the healer be open to new and novel ideas and concepts.

The individual who wishes to be a healer should first be educated by an experienced and competent healing instructor, such as Barbara or Helen. I also endorse the work of Rolf Steiner at the Snow Lion Center in Switzerland (another of Barbara's first-generation students, a very talented healer and instructor).

It is important to remember that not all patients are destined to be healed by any therapy or modality. This is because they may have their illness as part of their earthly experience or even their way out of this incarnation. Part of the main role of the healer is therefore to recognize this and to respond accordingly by helping them cope with their illness or transition but not trying to heal them. Watch the ego in this instance, it will make you have the desire to be the best healer on the planet and want to heal them. You will ultimately fail in this respect. Also, be aware of the patient that comes to you after a long list of healers have failed them. Again, watch the ego. If twenty healers cannot heal a patient, maybe it's in their life plan to experience this. Maybe they are using the illness to gain attention! The healer has to be vigilant at all times.

Although I advise against using this book as an instructional healing text, I expect that some readers will do just that. If this is the case, I accept no responsibility for the results, positive or negative.

An experienced healer will be aware of some of the expectations of a patient, and in some instances, their desperation and how persuasive this can be. But even the experienced healer can be caught out. In this respect, I offer the following advice.

- Observe the patient physically and energetically
- Communicate with their Guide and helpers
- Talk to them about what's happening to them:
    - Physically
    - Mentally
    - In relationships
    - In work
    - Their past
- Watch your ego
- Respect the patient
- Do not abuse your position, i.e.,
    - Do not suggest they need five appointments when one will do
    - Do not create financial dependence with a patient
    - Do not allow a patient to be dependent upon you for their well-being
- Respect yourself
- Know when you can't help them
- Don't be persuaded to help when you can't
- Be careful in how you word or explain that which you see or perceive (or intuit)
- Be caring
- DO NOT TAKE ON THEIR ISSUES OR RESPONSIBILITY FOR THEIR PROBLEMS

I hope you, dear reader, found this book an interesting illustration of what other healing techniques/ modalities are available and how in some instances they can be used.

Remember, being a healer is being of service. It is both an honor and a great responsibility.

Tread wisely and you will be successful.

*Guy Needler*
*23rd September 2019*

# Recommended Reading


Brennan, Barbara. *Hands of Light* (Bantam Books, Transworld Publishers a division of the Random House Group); Reissue edition (1 Feb. 1990).

Brennan, Barbara. *Light Emerging: The Journey of Personal Healing* (Bantam Books, Transworld Publishers a division of the Random House Group); 1st edition (1 Nov. 1993).

Thesenga, Susan (together with Eva Pierrakos, and Asha Greer, Illustrator). *The Undefended Self: Living the Pathwork* (Pathwork Press); 3rd edition (November 3, 2017).

Pierrakos, Eva, Thesenga, Donovan (editor): *Fear No Evil: The Pathwork Method of Transforming the Lower Self* (Pathwork Press); Revised edition (July 13, 2018).

Pierrakos, Eva, and Donovan Thesenga (editor). *Surrender to God Within: Pathwork at the Soul Level* (Pathwork Press) (November 26, 2013).

# Glossary

**Akashic Records**—An eternal past, present, and future record of each humankind's actions and subsequent evolution.

**Ascended Master**—An entity or being that has moved beyond the need to incarnate in a particular evolutionary cycle. Specifically, we can relate to the evolutionary cycle that we are in currently as an example. An Ascended Master is not necessarily one that has a record of incarnation within the Earth environment.

**The Animal Aspect**—An Aspect whose TES has a lower sentient content than human TES's. It can evolve beyond its TES. When it does so it detaches itself from the TES and seeks out a human TES of an evolutionary level (frequency of domicile) that is consistent with its self and negotiates integration and subsequent elevation to human status.

**Aspect**—An Aspect is a smaller part of the TES that is used to experience the minute detail of the environments within the multiverse. It is used to experience the lowest frequencies of the multiverse presented by the physical universe through the process of incarnation. A maximum of twelve Aspects can be projected by the TES at any one time.

**Being**—An individualized unit of sentience that has developed independently by the function of similar, same, or sympathetic energy/ies collecting together and evolving over a period.

**Chakra**—An energy center in the human body.

**Core Star meditations**—A method of meditation focused upon understanding one's life plan/task or reason for incarnation through accessing our greater beingness via the Hara or Core Star).

**Core Star**—The point or location of the division of sentience and energy of the incarnate Aspect within the human vehicle. The energy used to animate the human vehicle coalesces in the Tan Tien (located two inches below the navel and three inches in toward the center of the body) with the sentience coalescing in the Soul Seat (located close the point where the front and rear aspects of the heart chakras are joined or located, close to the thymus). The Core Star is often mistaken for the Tan Tien as it is so close to the Core Star. The Core Star is positioned two inches (5 cm) above the navel (belly button) and three inches (7.5 cm) in toward the center of the human vehicle from the navel.

**Dimensiate**—An effect of being pan dimensional (across many dimensions simultaneously).

**DNA**—Deoxyribonucleic acid Dysfunction—out of specification functionality Energy levels—the distance between each level that is consistent with the difference between the frequencies in the human auric levels.

**Dualistic**—A condition where two realities are in existence concurrently due to the possibility of an alternative reality being created when a choice of two directions is available.

**Entity**—An individualized unit of sentience given a body of energy/ies by the division of sentience away from a higher entity, by that higher entity.

**Event Space**—An area or volume of space within me that exists as a parallel function of that space. It is space overlapping space or space within and without a space. Everything exists in terms of events and not in terms of time. Event Space can be duplicated or parallelized because the creation of a new Event Space is the result of collective or individualized desire and is usually one of a number of possibilities or probabilities that are aligned to the current Event Space and Event Stream (see below). Event Space expands and contracts as necessary within its own space. When a single entity through its desires, intentions, thoughts, and actions does something on its own, it may be capable of creating an Event Space local to itself. However, in the event that the actions of the entity are enough to make other entities change their own ideas, desires, intentions, thoughts, behaviors, and actions, then it can invoke a new Event Space via collective desire.

**Experiential Vocabulary**—The total memory set of a particular incarnation. That being, the audible, visual, tangible (the full sensory experience) that an aspect or soul experiences during its current incarnation that is used to translate what is experienced in the energetic if there is no direct energetic experiential content available.

**Frequential Plane**—A singular sequential frequency.

**Frequential**—Sequentially based frequencies in frequentic space.

**Frequentially**—Sequentially based frequencies in frequentic (multifrequency) space.

**Frequentic**—Multifrequency space.

**God Head**—The Hindu word/descriptor for the TES.

**Hara Line**—The energetic link from the True Energetic Self (TES) to the incarnate vehicle. It links the Aspect projected into the human vehicle with the vehicle and the frequencies associated with the physical universe. It is the power and communication source of the human vehicle. The Hara Line is positioned in the center of the human form from the center of the top of the head, splitting into two at the Tan Tien and continuing earthward down the legs.

**Higher Self**—A spiritual word/descriptor for the TES.

**Hot Swop**—A computer peripheral term used to describe the removal or plugging in of a peripheral without the power being turned off. In the spiritual, this relates to the swopping in/out of a soul from/to a physical human body without the body needing to die or be born. This is sometimes called a walk-in.

**Human Aura**—The energy fields associated with the physical and astral components of the human body.

**Intelliate**—Intelligence-based communication.

**Lossy**—A computer term used to describe a conversion function that results in a reduction of some sort due to an either incorrect conversion factor or a specific function of the process used. Certain "losses" are sometimes considered acceptable, but this is only the case where the output is not critical, i.e., converting an image to JPEG is a lossy conversion function.

**OM**—Energy-based beings not indigenous to Earth.

**Omniciate**—Omniscience-based communication.

**Omnifunctional**—To be able to operate, as if in an individualized way, within all environments, spaces, and events, irrespective of structural conditions and parallelized versions, concurrently.

**Omnipresent**—To be located within all environments, spaces, and events, irrespective of structural conditions and parallelized versions concurrently.

**Omniscient**—To be focused within one's sentience that is located within all environments, spaces, and events, irrespective of structural conditions and parallelized versions concurrently.

**Over Soul**—The Quantum Healing Hypnosis Technique (QHHT) word/descriptor for the TES. QHHT was a hypnosis-based healing technique taught by Dolores Cannon.

**Polyomniscient**—A multiple aspect of Omniscience. A condition that will be achieved by The Origin as it expands into those areas of itself that are beyond its current area of sentient self-awareness.

**Primary Incarnation**—A descriptor for the incarnate functionality of an Aspect if a secondary incarnation is employed.

**Quadrulistic**—A condition where four realities are in existence concurrently due to the possibility of alternative realities being created when a choice of four directions is available.

**Readings or Reader**—Acting as a medium for a client who wants to know more information about themselves from spirit, but is not able to ask for themselves during meditation or any other means. A "Medium" gives a "Reading."

**RNA**—Ribonucleic acid Simulacrum—similar or in the same likeness.

**Secondary Incarnation**—A descriptor for the incarnate functionality of an Aspect that uses a significant percentage of its sentient energies to have an incarnation in a lower frequency within the physical universe. This is not a Shard but an incarnation within an incarnation because the Aspect in the primary incarnation continues while the secondary incarnation is in action. In the event that the Primary incarnation is placed in stasis for the duration of the secondary incarnation the primary incarnation will re-commence once the secondary incarnation is finished.

**Self-Realization**—The function of being in full command of all our faculties as an energetic being while in the physical.

**Sentiate**—Sentience-based communication.

**Shard**—A Shard is a smaller part of the Aspect that is used to experience the minute detail of the environments within the multiverse. It is also used to experience the lowest frequencies of the multiverse presented by the physical universe through the process of incarnation. As with the TES a maximum of twelve Shards can be projected by the Aspect at any one time.

**The Silver Cord**—The connection between the incarnate vehicle and the Aspect or Soul projected into it. Some individuals with enhanced ability to communicate with spirit have two silver cords.

**Soul Seat**—This is where the sentience of the Aspect resides. It is the personality of what we are, as a projected Aspect of our TES; "it is our sentience." Its position is close to where the front and rear Aspects of the heart chakra join, close to the thymus.

**Soul**—The Christian and spiritual word/descriptor for the Aspect or Shard. The Soul is considered to be individualized in totality and not part of a larger being. It is also generally related with the human body and no other incarnate vehicles.

**The Source Entity**—what we call God, the creator of our multiverse.

**Spaced out**—A term I used to describe being close to fainting.

**Spirituo-physical**—The level where the gross physical and energetic/ spiritual frequency levels meet and mix.

**Sub Incarnation**—A descriptor for the incarnate functionality of a Shard.

**Tan Tien**—This is where the energy of the Aspect spreads out into the energy network that contains the energy template and the chakras. It ends up being a focus of tremendous energy. It is positioned two inches (5 cm) below the navel (belly button) and three inches (7.5 cm) in toward the center of the human vehicle from the navel.

**Trilistic**—A condition where three realities are in existence concurrently due to the possibility of alternative realities being created when a choice of three directions is available.

**True Energetic Self**—(TES) what we truly are, an entity of pure sentience with a given or commandeered body of energy.

**Walk-In**—The swapping in and out (one for another) of Aspects (souls) within a single incarnate vehicle. There are many variations upon this theme.

**Where the TES Exists**—The TES exists in more than one place within the multiverse. It exists in the frequency associated with its evolutionary stasis and under evolutionary tension (see *The Origin Speaks*). Where it would have been had it not been in evolutionary stasis, and just evolved without using incarnation as an accelerant. And, where it would have been once the evolutionary tension is released.

# About the Author

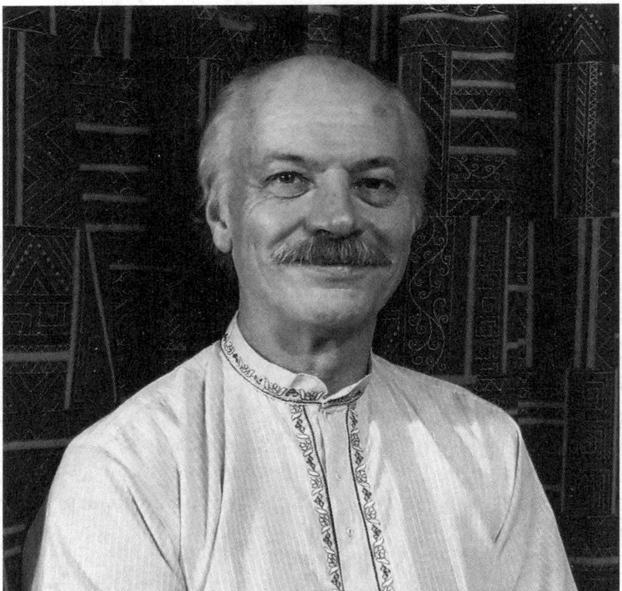

Guy Needler MBA, MSc, CEng, MIET, MCMA initially trained as a mechanical engineer and quickly progressed on to be a chartered electrical and electronics engineer. However, throughout this earthly training he was always aware of the greater reality being around him, catching glimpses of the worlds of spirit. This resulted in a period from his teenage to early twenties where he reveled in the spiritual texts of the day and meditated intensively. Being subsequently told by his guides to focus on his earthly contribution for a period he scaled back the intensity of spiritual work until his late thirties where he was re-awakened to his spiritual roles. The next six years saw him gaining his Reiki Master and a four year commitment to learn energy and vibrational therapy techniques from a direct student of the Barbara Brennan School of HealingTM, which also included a personal development undertaking (including psychotherapy) as a course prerequisite using the PathworkTM methodology described by Susan Thesenga with further methodologies by Donovan Thesenga, John and Eva Pierrakos. His training and experience in energy based therapies have resulted in him being a member of the Complementary Medical Association (MCMA).

Along with his healing abilities his spiritual associations include being able to channel information from spirit including constant contact with other entities within our multi-verse and his higher self and guides. It is the channeling that has resulted in "The History of God" and is producing further work.

As a method of grounding Guy practices and teaches Aikido. He is a 6th Dan National Coach with 38 years experience and is currently working on the use of spiritual energy within the physical side of the art.

Guy welcomes questions on the subject of spiritual physics and who and what God is.

# If you liked this book, you might also like:

*Sleep Magic*
by Voctoria Pendragon
*The Sleeping Phoenix*
by Victoria Pendragon
*Being In A Body*
by Victoria Pendragon
*Divine Gifts of Healing*
by Cat Baldwin
*A Small Book of Comfort*
by Lyn Willmott
*The Master of Everything*
by James Nussbaumer
*Who Catharted*
by Blair Styra